HOW THE LIGHT COMES IN

A memoir of hope and healing on the path with anxiety.

Carlee J. Hansen

© 2022 Carlee J. Hansen

All rights reserved. No portion of this book may be reproduced or distributed in any form or by any means without expressed, written consent from the publisher.

Printed by KDP, an Amazon.com Company

Library of Congress Cataloging-in-Publication Data
Hansen, Carlee J, 1982-
How the Light Comes In: A memoir of hope and healing on the path with anxiety.
ISBN-13: 978-0-578-28143-8

To all who are fighting their own silent battle.

Fight on.

CONTENTS

	Introduction	1
1	In the Beginning	7
2	Seeking Help	15
3	Therapy	17
4	Tools	25
5	Work	35
6	Medical Help	43
7	A Long December	57
8	Stigma	65
9	Sacred Things	69
10	Where are you, God?	77
11	Church	85
12	Small and Simple	89
13	Chasing Perfection	91
14	Exposure	95
15	2020	99
16	Recovery	107
17	The Dance	113
18	Final Thoughts	117
19	Afterword	123
	Acknowledgements	127

INTRODUCTION

Every year in early to mid-July, most of Northern Utah participates in a celebration of our pioneer heritage. How do we do this? Well, how all people celebrate momentous occasions in their lives – with fireworks; Weber State University puts on a fantastic spectacular of lights and sound as all of us gather on the grass/illegally park to watch the show. It is a great time for families to gather and to spend a night celebrating our statehood.

Our little family has a tradition of going to this firework show each year; we load up our oversized truck with lawn chairs and snacks and make our way to the parking lot of a grocery store that is in close proximity to the school and nestle in amongst the other cars. We always feel like we have a bit of an advantage because rather than having to park and find a spot to sit, our parking stall *is* our spot to sit. We climb into the back of our truck and set up our chairs like the class act we always pretend to be and watch as hundreds of families drag coolers and chairs (and children) for blocks, hoping for a comfortable destination with a view.

I have fond memories of this night – being together and laughing and watching our kids try to dance or play charades. I remember one particular year like it was yesterday... and I can't tell you a single thing about the actual fireworks because of a conversation that was started with my husband before the show began.

I made mention the watch that I was wearing was a little too snug on my wrist and he asked the simplest of questions: "Do you have extra links at home that we could add to it?"

"I don't know. Maybe."

And that was all it took. I started thinking about whether I did have extra watch links at home and if I did, where they would be located. I mentally searched through my entire jewelry case, looking for remnants of rose gold and wondering if they were tucked away somewhere. I started wondering if maybe I kept the original box my watch came in and if maybe I had kept the links in there, or if I had kept the watch box at all. I became consumed with needing to know if I had extra links at home, thinking of nothing else and barely being able to stay sitting at that firework show for need to know what I was dealing with. *Did I have extra links at home?!*

As soon as we pulled into the driveway, I made my way (read: nearly pushed my kids over) up to my room to scour all the places that said links would be and you know what? There weren't any. Anywhere. And I felt so much better.

This is the part of the story where some of you may get a bewildered look on your face and wonder what just happened. "Didn't you *want* the links? Weren't you disappointed in not finding them? What is the point of this whole story?"

In short: yes, I did want the watch links because it would have saved me time and money, not having to reorder some from the watch manufacturer; that would have been great. But in truth, it wasn't the watch links I was after; it was closure. I needed to know the answer, good or bad, have or not have, about the links. I needed to not be in limbo. Once I finally knew there were no links to be found, my mind could rest and move on to other worries.

And in case you haven't guessed by this point, I have a lot of them.

I suppose there have been signs my whole life that I had high-functioning anxiety; that's what my therapist called it and to be called high-functioning *anything* seemed like a compliment so I thought I had better include it here as a resume builder. Despite categorizing myself as a chronic "worrier" at a fairly young age (is it weird to be concerned about your 401k in sixth grade?), I never really came face-to-face with this governing part of my personality until I was in my 30s – you know, when worries about yourself turn to worries about mortgages and careers and aging parents and your kids' future, all the really lightweight stuff.

Then, in my mid-30s, I had an experience that forever changed my perspective on mental health and self-care and God and family and all the things. In mid-December of 2018, I had my first full-blown panic attack. I'll write more about this as we move forward but for now, suffice it to say this experience showed me how dark anxiety can be when you don't find ways to recognize it and work through it and heal; I'm still working on that and likely will for the rest of my life.

So why write about this? Why tell everyone my dark secrets? Because writing is part of *my* process and on the small chance that reading is part of yours, here I am.

I wrote a book previously, titled "Peas are Gross", and it was exactly what everyone expected from me; a life-long subscriber to the mantra that humor can fix anything, it was (is – still available on Amazon, wink, wink) a satirical look at life and it's nuances like work and exercise and raising kids and dating (not necessarily in that order). I always joke that it belongs in every gas station/restaurant on Route 66, right next to the cowboy poetry.

"Peas are Gross" was a comfortable piece for me because humor is my weapon of choice; it is how I have always attacked life and is still my go-to when things get hairy. Joy is my most sacred feeling and being able to bring that to the table (even in a gas station diner) on occasion is a most fulfilling calling. I love that I come from funny stock who make me take life less seriously at times – it is truly my greatest blessing.

This book is not that. While I do hope you will find some humor in these pages, I hope you also know this book comes from a very different place in my heart – one that most people haven't been privy to in my lifetime.

This book isn't written as any sort of medical diagnosis; in fact, you probably shouldn't even consider it a self-help guide because I am in no way a doctor or even an expert in diagnosing or recognizing anxiety and depression. (If you happen to find this book in any sort of section at a book store that may allude to it being medically-charged or self-help, I need you to do two things: first, take a picture of you with my book in a book store because I promise I'll need proof that a book store wanted to try and sell my thoughts on things. Yay! I've made it! Second, tell a manager immediately that this book has been misclassified and really belongs in the "thoughts on stuff" section of the store.)

The only real qualification I have that allows me to tell you about anything related to anxiety and depression is this: I lived it.

This will not perfectly describe your battle with anxiety nor the one that your closest confidante is going through. It is my un-professional opinion that these things manifest themselves differently in each of us.

What this book will tell you is that this complicated and prevalent human frailty is real. This book outlines my very personal relationship with anxiety and all she has to bring to the table. I expose the jugular and talk about my very real (albeit unfounded) worries and the crisis of faith it triggered in my own life. Most importantly, I will tell you about healing. Not the kind of healing brought on by pills or therapists (although I will talk about those and can I get a pre-emptive "hallelujah" for the role that both played in my recovery), but the kind of healing that comes from work and meditation and prayer and self-discovery.

This struggle has been so personal and so wrenching for me, as it is for thousands of men and women navigating these same rough waters. But I've also grown and changed in ways that couldn't have come about in any other way. And for those of you taking wave after wave, unable to come up for air, I hope this piece of me will supply the smallest amount hope and that you will always know there is room in my raft if you need; we can ride out the storm together.

IN THE BEGINNING

I still look around every day and ask myself this question: what happened here? I think this is a commonality amongst anyone who has had some sort of life-changing event take them by surprise: the death of a loved one, a friendship that suddenly spirals into nothingness, the loss of a job; there are just things that happen in our lives that cause us to sit up in the morning, reflect on the previous day or week or month and leave us in a metal stupor.

To be honest, I don't know what happened. There were no major events that transpired that would have left me feeling helpless and emotionally wrecked, no warning, no cause. At the same time, there were a million little things I had dealt with for so long that I think my brain (and quite possibly my soul) decided to initiate a protest and just shut down.

Angst is something I'm used to; a born worrier, I've spent most of my adult life nervous. I worry about bills and jobs and schedules and... sound familiar? Maybe because that's called adulting. We *all* worry about those things. I realize now that maybe my worry was excessive when my mind automatically went to the worst-case scenario for everything; if I saw a report about a school shooting, I would make a plan about what I would do if my kids' school were under attack. Like a REAL plan in my head. A normal person may think about it for a minute and write off the incident as a tragic happenstance, but not me. I did this with everything from winter storm warnings to nuclear negotiations with North Korea. I had a "bail-out" plan for everything.

The weird part is that I didn't do all this planning inside a nuclear bunker like the crazies I had pitied on television. I worried while I made dinner and drove my kids to gymnastics and while I took a shower. I planned birthday parties and trips to Disney and mowed the lawn, all while plotting my next move. My point is that I functioned through all of it and frankly, probably appeared amazingly carefree to the people around me as I made every attempt to stay busy and engaged; inside, I was reeling. To most people, I appeared put-together (their words, certainly not mine) and involved. After all, what could I have to worry about?

Shy of never getting asked to my high school prom and an occasional argument with my insurance company, my problems were minimal. I grew up in a middle-class neighborhood and rode bikes with my friends. I had two parents in our home who worked hard and loved harder, and we never lacked for what we needed. I got good grades and played sports and spent a lot of weekends changing from my soccer uniform into a dress for my piano recital, all in the back seat of our family van. I went to college on scholarship and did all the fun things you do in college – well, that *we* do in college; did I mention that I grew up in Utah? Normally, I don't know that location would matter in this discussion but trust me, it's a point of importance.

Before you panic, you have not been duped into reading some anti-establishment rhetoric nor am I about to tell you how my beliefs and cultural surroundings have ruined my life. This is not *that* book and I'm not going to say that, because truthfully, they haven't. In fact, my membership and subsequent full-time activity in The Church of Jesus Christ of Latter-Day Saints has been the only consistent part of my life over the past 30 years and as a self-proclaimed worrier, you can imagine that consistency is something I hold dear. I am a believer. I always have been, and I pray I always will be.

What I *am* saying is that Utah, albeit beautiful, can have a nasty underbelly culturally, one that expects a lot out of its people. While we are known for our mountains and our national parks and our clean-living (except for the winter smog – can we all just agree to get it together and do something about this??!), internally we are also known for our chase for perfection - economically, mentally and spiritually. My religious convictions mandate a focus on the eventual and eternal, a focus that can make living in and appreciating the "now" fairly difficult. As the unofficial DIY capital of North America (a self-inflicted title, I don't know that there really is a contest for this), the pressure can feel real to do everything and be everything and make everything, all while having your spiritual life put together and having great hair. We are a resourceful people, for sure, but these lofty expectations weigh heavily on a good portion of women, a fact I've really come to recognize over the past few years.

I've never been one to consciously feel like I needed to keep up with the Joneses. Generally speaking, I don't think I've ever even *liked* the Joneses. But our subconscious can be a tricky beast and you never know what it's going to tell you. In early December 2018, mine told me that I was beyond tired and as I wrapped up several important and long-standing tasks/assignments in my life, my mind decided to take a much-needed sabbatical. I didn't feel it coming on; there weren't warning signs except for an increasing amount of apathy and a shortened temper (sorry kids and husband). Short of that, life, my life, was normal on a Saturday… and then not on a Sunday.

We had just returned from a weekend stay in Park City and I was feeling particularly somber. I had been having back problems for several weeks and had spent a good portion of the weekend in our hotel room with heat therapy. Regardless, we had a great time as a family; our annual Park City trip is something I look forward to all year and I treasure the time I get to be with my parents and family. I always go home feeling lifted and laughed out and grateful.

When we arrived home that evening, I found myself in a full panic attack. I had never had a panic attack before, so I was unsure of what was happening other than incoherent sobs and an increased heartrate for longer than I was comfortable. I've since learned that panic attacks are generally sudden and are accompanied by feelings of fear or dread and can be escorted by a myriad of physical responses including increased pulse, breathlessness, weak muscles, dizziness – the list goes on like a bad prescription commercial. But at the time, I felt weak and scared and lost for no apparent reason. It was not my best look.

I decided to take a hot bath, hoping the heat would calm my nerves, but it was no use. I sobbed and sobbed and found myself begging God not to let me die. Important note of clarification here: I was not sick. I had not been issued a terminal diagnosis; I didn't even have a common cold. I wasn't being dramatic nor feeling sorry for myself. I honestly felt in my head and in my soul that these moments were going to be my last on Earth. This was it. It was over.

The tricky thing about staring down death in your mind is that it doesn't end; there is no point that comes where your conscious mind can say, "See, we are ok. We beat that scary thing. Good work. Let's move on," because there was nothing to *beat* in the first place. My mind was sure I was going to die and there was no resolution to that. And that is where it all began.

If I would have written down what anxiety felt like prior to having panic attacks, I would have said something about worry along with a tinge of excitement or anticipation about an upcoming event. All-in-all, that seems like a normal human reaction to change or something unexpected making an appearance in your life.

Without trying to sound melodramatic, I'd now define actual anxiety as something totally different; words like "crippling" and "repetitive" and "cloudy" are now included along with feelings of angst and nausea and despair, coupled with fear and sadness. The worst part (for me) is the complete inability to control these emotions or to logically wash them away. Minutes in this place feel like hours as sleep evades, appetite disappears, and your sense of control completely vanishes. Nothing feels familiar or safe and even as a full-grown adult, that is terrifying.

I spent the next couple of days in a stupor; afraid of my impending death, I didn't sleep because that's how death gets you, right? If I just didn't sleep, I could control my dying. I know this thought process sounds completely irrational, and I'll admit it was. But please remember that when these 'irrational' thoughts are taking place in the middle of panic and anxiety, they are as real as the sky is blue.

Now seems like a good time to talk a little bit about the physiology of my panic and anxiety because it helped me to understand what was going on in my brain and why I felt so out of control. As with the other 4,000 times in this book I will warn you about this, I am not a doctor, nor do I play one on tv. But research was a huge part of my healing and I think some of the things I found out may be useful here. Again, I can only discuss what was happening with *me* in hopes it will spark a desire to find out what may be happening physiologically with you, not as a recommendation or any sort of diagnosis – that is way above my pay grade. As you read, you will clearly see I am not a doctor and may use terms like "thingy" in my explanations.

There are two parts of the brain that are seriously affected during a panic attack and during the subsequent anxiety. The front part of the brain processes logic and allows for rational thinking while the back part of the brain houses our adrenaline – our fight or flight response – and is the part of our brain that gets all crazy when we are panicked. The interesting thing I discovered is that these two parts of the brain cannot be fully "on" at the same time, and for good reason. When we are truly feeling threatened, truly in fight or flight mode, there is nothing rational about survival; we do whatever is necessary to get out of that situation and return our brain and body to homeostasis (that's a big word I learned for "normal"). This is why as women, we are always told to "have a plan" for a variety of dangerous situations we could find ourselves in; if you wait until you are in it, it likely won't turn out well.

Another key factor in *my* anxiety is something called intrusive thinking; this part of my cognition is exactly what it sounds like – a weird second-cousin who comes to stay and won't ever leave. (I actually have never experienced this. People don't stay with me – something about too many rules? Go figure.) Once a thought pops into my head, it stays until there is some form of concrete resolution. Intrusive thinking is a pig because the thoughts that come into my mind are front and center, on constant repeat; if the thought would camp somewhere in the recesses of my mind, it wouldn't be that big of a deal because all of my pressing issues would be looked at and addressed once a day and I could live a normal life. With intrusive thinking, however, that thought stays right at the front of my mind until it is resolved. I think about a bill until it is paid or resolved, a meeting until it concludes, a watch link until it is found. I fixate on these thoughts until they can be resolved with nearly indisputable evidence. You do not want to be around when I lose something… or for the 15 days after.

I want to be very clear that I had no idea this was a "thing", a diagnosis, until I had lived with it for 36 years. I just thought when people talked about worry that this feeling of unsettled angst was what they were referring to. I know that sounds crazy but my version of worry was all I knew so that became my point of reference. Only after visiting an intuitive therapist for about 12 seconds did he recognize this off-shoot of obsessive-compulsive disorder in me and let me know that my way of thinking was, in fact, a big "thing" and was probably one of the many factors leading to my panic attacks.

It's funny, I read through all of this now and piece together everything that led up to my panic attack and it all makes perfect sense — the obsession and the pressure and the way I handled worry were a clear path to a breakdown in my bathtub. But it wasn't weird or hard for me until it was too much. That's the tricky part about anxiety and panic - it truly is all in your head; thoughts and memories and worries continue to process in the depths of your mind until they decide to creep into the light and remind you that they are still there and finally ready to be dealt with. And once they manifest in the form of anxiety, you have no choice but to deal with them, straight on, in one way or another.

It is critical to note that the understanding of what was happening in my head came after a trek down a long and painful path. If someone had tried to explain the physiology of this to me or to rationalize me through my situation while I was in the throes of it, it wouldn't have mattered. In fact, several well-meaning family members and doctors and emergency room attendants confirmed over and over that I was a healthy, living, breathing person and had nothing to worry about, and I still had the utmost confidence in my impending doom. My head told me different and my heart was so very sad at the time, I was sure they had all missed something and I *knew* different.

All it took was a minute to go from my 'normal' self to a panic-stricken mess. One single minute for my brain to decide I hadn't been a very good comrade for a very long time and it was going on a break. So, it decided to fixate on the one thing that had no concrete resolution — death — and put it on repeat, figuring that specific track ought to keep me busy for a while. And it did.

SEEKING HELP

I wish at this point in my story, I could say that I sought help through the channels that most faith-based stories revel in. Believe me, I prayed. I prayed and I sobbed, a topic I'll discuss more in a later chapter but suffice it for now to say, things in that department weren't going as I hoped.

As I sat in my living room, I did what all wise people having a nervous breakdown should do: I started Googling. (If it isn't abundantly clear, that was thick, *thick* sarcasm. When you are sick, stay off the internet. It only makes things worse.) First it was symptoms, although searching "I feel like I'm going to die" is not a rabbit hole you want to go down, trust me. Then it rapidly turned into a shotgun approach to simply "feeling better" which yielded 86,000 search results, and those were only the ones that included essential oils.

I spoke with my mom about how I was feeling and after some encouragement, my online searches quickly migrated from symptomatic to solutions-based. She and I had joked previously about how my worries were so thick that maybe I should talk to someone, a professional someone, and get them sorted out. This time though, it didn't feel like it was in jest. I needed help.

Therapy seemed like a good starting point for me; I hadn't even considered medication or other types of intervention because those were for "other people". In my naiveite, I figured that one hour-long session with a professional listener should clear my brain and I'd be able to move forward. Because that's how it worked. Again, on tv.

I've always been a rule-follower (surprise!) so I knew that whatever a therapist told me to do, I'd do it. My can-do attitude was strengthened by the fact that I had never felt so sad or afraid in my life; if my new therapist told me drinking 12 oz of dog urine every day would clear up my current state, I'd import the drink from China. I was that desperate for help.

I learned quickly that you physically *can* reach a point where you would do anything to get out of your own head; what that means for each of us is different and I still consider myself fortunate that the furthest my head went during this initial process was therapy and not to something more sinister. I am constantly thinking about those who are suffering and so desperate to heal that they consider taking drastic measures to end it all. I always wondered why victims of suicide couldn't be stronger and always questioned, "how bad could it really be?" but that was only because I didn't understand the dark. Now that I've seen those murky recesses of my own mind, I'll forever be grateful that therapy is where I turned first and I was able to receive respite before it was too late.

THERAPY

I want to start this section with total transparency: I never believed in therapy. Ok, maybe that is not true. I figured there were some super "messed up" people who probably needed therapy to recover from childhood trauma but I didn't believe in it in the general sense, in the sense it would ever apply to me. In fact, I always pitied the people who felt like they had to turn to a stranger to get their feelings verbalized and understood.

Important side note here: I'm fully aware that my pre-panic life is starting to make me sound like an emotionally-stunted alien with little empathy or insight; I've alluded to the fact that I didn't understand why people couldn't just pull up on their boot straps and get to work. It's not that I wasn't empathetic, I just had no frame of reference. The way we solved issues in my family *was* to pull up on our boot straps and get to work. We felt all the things, but we certainly didn't wallow. I had a really loving and understanding family growing up so it never even crossed my mind to turn to anyone besides my parents, my brother or, eventually, my husband, when things got difficult. Therapy wasn't for people like me with emotional outlets and incoming love and seemingly perfect support. At least I didn't think it was.

So, when the time came that I knew in the most guttural sense that I needed to schedule time to talk to a therapist, I was terrified. I had no childhood trauma to address (with the exception of my brother sitting on my chest and threatening to drop spit on my face – now who has the last laugh, bro? I'm telling the world on you, not just mom.) and I certainly had no interest in laying on anyone's couch and looking at Rorschach diagrams to find the true meaning of life. Despite my ill-conceived notions about therapy, I knew it was what I had to do.

There are thousands and thousands of resources available to people seeking therapy. There are online directories of therapists specializing in anxiety, location-based directories where you can find a therapist within six blocks of your house, even lists of therapists who will offer their services via email so you don't have to be humiliated (if that's your worry) about talking to someone face-to-face. So, believe me when I say me finding my particular therapist was nothing short of God showing me that He had not, in fact, left my side.

I found one of those directories that they tout on the radio and I am here to testify that searching for a therapist based solely on their profile picture is far more intimidating than any dating site – the stakes feel much, much higher when you are looking for someone to save your mental health and not just take you to dinner. Nearly all of the therapists who were listed in my area looked nice and professional and were happy to take insurance, so I scrolled… and scrolled… and stopped at a nice-looking gentleman who had two very important characteristics: first, he looked older than me. I know that sounds completely trite but it would have been extremely difficult for me to visit a therapist only to find out that I graduated the same year as their much older sister. This happened to me at an ENT once and it is weird talking about junior high with someone as they scope your throat. It also reassured me that when I sat down in his office, he wouldn't be breaking the seal on his "Therapy 101" book, but had some years of experience.

Second, he looked… normal. Most people probably don't think about these things but in my already fragile mental state, I didn't want to sit cross-legged on a rug while hemp burned in the background and I aligned my chakras, NOR did I want someone telling me how smart they were under the guise of it being "therapy". I'm fully aware that first impressions are a terrible platform to make decisions on (Don't @ me. I've been chubby my whole life and have been wrongfully judged since I was three, so I get it) but when all I had to go off of was a picture and a standard "about me" questionnaire, I had to do what I had to do.

After a lengthy pep-talk in my living room ("It's ok. People do this. If you hate it, you can leave. His secretary probably won't call you back anyway."), I called. Surprisingly enough, my call went to voicemail. HIS voicemail. Like a personal voicemail. (To be fair, I figured I would not likely speak to a doctor on the first try but I had never done this and I assumed there would be a secretary who asked me to rate my craziness or screen me or something… but not personal voicemail.)

I'm going to go ahead and tell you what that voicemail sounded like, just in case you are ever considering calling a therapist and are terrified and afraid you are going to sound stupid. This, my good reader, is hard evidence that no matter what you say, you will never sound *this* stupid. This should give you some solace. You're welcome.

Carlee: Um yeah, hi. I am calling because you are a therapist. And I think I need one. I mean maybe I don't, but I think so. And you are one. And your picture is nice. I mean you seem nice. Like from your picture. And now your voicemail. So, you are probably busy, because you are nice. So yeah, I think I need… see, I'm having a panic attack. I mean not now, well sort of now but mostly before. And I think it is panic? That's what Google says. But I don't know. This has never happened before. I'm fine, but I'm scared. But not really fine or I guess I wouldn't be calling. Can you please call me back? Please?

Machine: If you are satisfied with your message...

Heck no I wasn't satisfied with my message! But I knew the likelihood of me re-recording that message and it being even *slightly* more coherent than that was slim, so I went with it. He must have either been completely confused or had seen this movie before because not ten minutes later, I got a call back from Dr. G.

(Dr. G isn't an actual doctor in the title sense, and he would want to make sure I clarify that; he is a licensed therapist who specializes in anxiety. But for me, for only this purpose, a doctor is someone who saves your life and he most certainly aided in that. So, Dr. G, you are officially awarded an honorary doctorate from the "Carlee School of Hard Knocks". You earned it. Also, it would really be weird to continue to refer to him as CMHC G for the remainder of this chapter so I'm going with it to avoid confusion. Also, it lets me identify him without actually identifying him which is what all good books do, right?)

On the phone, Dr. G immediately made me feel less crazy, almost as if I hadn't just humiliated myself on his voicemail. He told me he got my message and he'd love to chat and that he had some free time the next day. The. Next. Day. Remember how we talked about intrusive thinking and about how once an issue presents itself, it doesn't leave without some concrete conclusion? This is the same with scheduling haircuts and therapy sessions; if I had to wait a month, I wouldn't have survived.

I tell you the gory details of this phone call not because it is fun to recount how dumb I was that first day, but because I want you to know that it is a process to even admit maybe things aren't ok... and that's ok. I had worked in marketing for over a decade, made thousands of calls to negotiate contract terms and worked with/for people whose cars cost more than my first house. And this was the most terrifying phone call I had ever made.

I felt like making that call was admitting defeat, that I couldn't take care of myself or my life anymore. In a sense, it was exactly that. I waved my white flag, albeit sheepishly, because I had no other option. I couldn't take care of myself or my life at that point, but it certainly didn't mean I would never be able to do it again. Calling a therapist felt HUGE only because I had never done it before, that's the bottom line. If I knew then what I know now about therapy, I would have done it years ago. Not because it's fun or because it solved all of my issues (it didn't), but because it gave me some additional insight into what it means to fully and completely trust someone else with 100% of the weirdest and scariest parts of me.

As I said earlier, I have an incredible family who have supported me through all of my journeyings. But no matter how close you are with your mom (and I am clooooooose), there are just certain things you would never say to her. Or maybe you would overanalyze it so it would come out just the right way and not hurt her feelings. Or you would only tell a partial truth because the other half sounds crazy, even in your head. This is absolutely no reflection on the mothers or siblings or dads or partners in our lives, it really is a mental defense we use to keep everything normal. We don't like seeing people upset or confused or frustrated with our feelings. And oddly enough, all of that reservation kind of goes away when you sit across from a total stranger (a trained total stranger, you guys. Don't do this at the bus station.), the *right* total stranger, and tell them how you are feeling, really feeling, about a whole cohort of topics. That is vulnerability in its truest form.

I'm not going to write that I think everyone should do "some sort" of therapy because I just don't think that is true. Therapy should be healing and the only way it is really effective is if you are lucky enough to find the right therapist with the right tools to address your very personal situation. Sounds like finding a needle in a haystack, right? Truthfully, it can be. Some people run the gamut of therapists, not only looking for a good personality fit but one who offers treatment solutions that are both applicable and feel possible in the midst of trauma. Many people are unable to find that right fit and quit therapy altogether, figuring it just isn't for them. It hasn't escaped me how fortunate I am to have thrown the dart and hit fairly close to the bullseye on the first throw. My sessions with Dr. G just felt right, despite the crying and complete confusion I felt at the time. And when you find the right therapist (if it ends up being something you need) and you start to process all the things, it is the most terrifying and yet freeing feeling on the planet.

Spoiler: the freeing part wins in the end.

The journey through therapy is not an easy one. In fact, after my first appointment with Dr. G, I got so wound up in everything that I ended up at another doctor's office – the medical kind. I woke up on the morning of my second therapy appointment and just could not get my head right. I was sick to my stomach and every muscle in my body ached as if I had just run a marathon (I imagine – I've never done that but I bet it really hurts). My heartbeat was crazy and I couldn't seem to focus. Surely, I had come down with something and needed to reschedule my appointment with Dr. G.

As the morning progressed, things got worse. Physically it got so bad that I had my mom (yeah, I'm a grown woman) drive me to our local health clinic to see a family practitioner - I was so sick that I didn't even care at that point who it was as long as they could help me with whatever was happening.

So much happened at that appointment that I will cover later but one thing came to light fairly quickly: I was apparently terrified of therapy. After speaking with the medical doctor about my symptoms and what I had been going through that morning, he quickly assessed that I was having a panic attack and that I had likely had one/multiple in my sleep the previous night. He asked if there was anything going on that I thought would make me anxious and I quickly shouted, "Yeah, I started therapy!" We both chuckled but it was true. I believe now that I had some sort of subconscious reaction to therapy and knowing I had to go back scared me to the point of another breakdown.

Fortunately, I pushed through the fear and did (eventually) re-schedule my second appointment with Dr. G. As we spoke, he challenged me to do several things I found ridiculous at the time but really were the foundation of my healing process; the first was to start writing things down.

TOOLS

Therapists have a tool bucket that is about as deep as anyone would ever need. A good therapist will find things that are natural for you to do and incorporate healing into those daily practices. I am a list-maker by trade and Dr. G encouraged me to start making a list of things I was grateful for. The items on the list could be simple but he recommended I do this when I could, preferably daily.

Gratitude

Gratitude seemed like such a simple concept that I was sure it would not work to ease my angst. I didn't feel ungrateful – I was very much aware of the good life I had led and was currently leading (present anxiety excepted, of course), so I didn't really understand how this would help me. Maybe you are the same? Sometimes answers can seem too simple to be helpful, like the people of Moses being asked to simply look at a staff and live; it just seemed too easy to be a legitimate answer to my problem. I'm sure if Dr. G had told me I needed to soak in a bath of warm red paint three times a day or drink that dog urine I referenced earlier, I would have taken him seriously but gratitude just seemed too elementary. But I started anyway.

After I started writing down a few things a day that I was grateful for (on a really ugly notebook filled with graphing paper – I was obviously taking this *vuuuury* seriously), I noticed a small shift. Keeping a list or a gratitude journal wasn't about making me more grateful, it was about distraction. It becomes pretty difficult to focus on your problems and feel-bads while you are thinking of all the ways you won the day or were blessed. Gratitude, much like service, is about stepping outside of yourself and letting go for a time, even a short time, each day.

Some days, my gratitude journal was awesome and filled with things like family and God and good friends. Other days, all I could find gratitude for was toilets and toothbrushes. Regardless of what made the list, taking the few minutes to reflect and write offered a change of perspective and sometimes, it was the spark that lit the fire for a good hour or night or, eventually, a good day.

I remember one night, sitting down to write in my journal and reflect. I had had a string of "toothbrush" kind of days and was determined to find something to be grateful for that couldn't be purchased in a pharmacy (this is a terrible joke from someone on anti-anxiety medications, but I can't help myself.). As I sat at my kitchen table, I thought about my life – my family and my home, my kids and my friends – and I very clearly remember thinking, "It can be enough." I felt a surge of peace come over me knowing if something were to happen to me, I had lived a life that could fill thousands of gratitude books and that is more than anyone could ask for. I also felt the calm reassurance that there were plenty of gratitude moments yet to be had and in that moment, I was ever so grateful. All I wrote in my journal that night was, "Life".

Whether you are struggling with anxiety or not, try to keep this gratitude thing in your back pocket. Don't feel the Insta-pressure to buy a fancy gratitude journal and a set of new pens UNLESS that will motivate you to use it; sometimes new stuff motivates me to start a journey (you should see how many pairs of running shoes I have) and if that will give you the push to start writing, save those pennies and get yourself a new notebook. But as a girl who started writing on literal graph paper, I can tell you that anything will do.

As you search for things to be grateful for, don't limit yourself to the majors. When I was really sick, I listed I was grateful for sweatpants. This was prior to Covid so me being in sweatpants was yet to become a social norm. But I specifically remember how that day, my sweatpants gave me the slightest sense of comfort; they were old and familiar and good. For even an instant, if sweatpants or blue jellybeans or toilet paper put on the correct way (always over, kids, always over) makes you feel at peace, it belongs in your journal. And if anyone questions that, you send them my way.

Exposure Therapy

The next thing Dr. G asked me to do was exposure work. Dr. G used cognitive behavioral therapy as a baseline for my treatment, implementing various strategies under that umbrella to aid in my healing. Cognitive behavioral therapy, in a sense, is all about changing the patterns of behavior that are associated with my anxiety in hopes of changing my thought process. I like to call it "prove your mind wrong" therapy but it doesn't sound as professional.

The crux of exposure therapy is basically doing things that make you uncomfortable in hopes of re-training your mind to think they aren't so bad. Eleanor Roosevelt once said, "You gain strength, courage and confidence by every experience in which you really stop to look fear in the face." I believe this is the essence of exposure therapy and it, my friends, truly is Work (notice that capital "W"). Not only do you have to recognize the discomfort when it is right in your face, you have to sit in it and let that discomfort take hold until it is gone. It is a terrifying notion to most people, but especially to anxiety pros. When we are placed in an uncomfortable situation, our "flight" senses take over the controls and prepare us to get out of Dodge immediately. Those senses aren't a small push, they are a tidal wave. So, sitting still while that tidal wave washes over you is a really daunting task.

Because explaining exposure therapy can be tricky, here is a quick example from my own therapy work that will hopefully explain it better than I can:

I have big issues with inconveniencing people. Big ones. I'm always early to things because I dread making people wait on me. I always did extra work on group projects so I for sure wouldn't be the one holding anyone back. I am constantly planning for the "just in case" so that I am not coming up short, and "bare minimum" is not in my vocabulary. So, Dr. G suggested that maybe one time, while I was at the grocery store, if the clerk asked me if I had found everything ok, I should say "no" … and then *wait* for them to either go find it or go and find the item myself while other people waited behind me in line. I am pretty sure I lost consciousness at the mere suggestion of doing this but I think it painted a very clear picture of what was expected of me; my job wasn't to worry about what other people thought or what I thought other people thought. My job was to stand there, in my discomfort, until the task was over. Doing this would help train my brain that discomfort did not equal death and despite being horribly uncomfortable, the discomfort would eventually end and life would move on.

Exposure therapy is exactly as raw and uncomfortable as it sounds. In fact, some therapists shy away from it because it becomes too daunting for a lot of patients to follow through with. Looking for ways to challenge your thinking isn't something you want on your daily "to-do" list. It also isn't a one-time cure-all. Exposure therapy is a continual process; every single time I start feeling uncomfortable or I start questioning myself and that loop starts, I have to take a step back and reassess what is triggering my anxiety, locate the root cause, and address it head on by facing the discomfort. I still practice this, even years later, in a variety of social situations from parties to one-on-one interactions with people.

Ironically, the interesting and valuable part about exposure therapy is the change that has taken place within myself after working *through* the discomfort that it brings. Being forced to reexamine and reevaluate what you think and believe can breathe life into you that you never knew existed. This type of therapy has helped me to realize how much of my life is based on perception and not actual fact, that my brain is pretty crafty about making situations into more than they actually are, and that it is absolutely ok to change my mind about a whole gamut of issues when the universe presents new truths to me on a platter.

Change can be terrifying, but none is quite as terrifying as changing your mind. But taking a step back to deconstruct my feelings and fears has been enlightening and given me perspective I never would have gained otherwise. The growth is in the challenge, and it is good.

Meditation

During my second session with Dr. G, we talked fairly extensively about insightfulness and meditation and the role it would play in my healing, yet another mindfulness practice I was not on-board with. If you haven't noticed the pattern as of yet, all of my preconceived notions about this, too, were about to be blown wide open.

I practiced meditation once in my life for about four days. I worked at a scout camp on Catalina Island one summer and a friend of mine was really into meditation. So, on a couple of evenings, I went with him and a couple of other people out to a platform by the bay and he taught us how to meditate. I was a terrible student. I laid there and listened to the water, and got the giggles, and started to nod off. I had zero self-control when it came to quiet self-reflection, a trait I continue to battle to this day.

At Dr. G's recommendation, I downloaded a couple of meditation apps that could help me in my practice. One was a guided meditation; for you novices like me, this is where they tell you what to relax and how to relax and what to think or not think about and basically talk you through your session. This did not work for me for a variety of reasons, the primary one being that my mind is a maze and thinking about one thing led to thoughts about sixty-five other things. I could not, for the life of me, turn off the connections and I ended up mentally exhausted at the end of each session.

The other type of app was more of a prompt-based mediation app; the program would give you an initial guide to the meditation for that day and then let you drift from there, playing soft music to accompany your thoughts. This also did not work for me. Generally during the soft music portion, I would pick up on a familiar beat and end up reciting lyrics to some REO Speedwagon song rather than focusing on my inner turmoil. It was distracting, but not helpful.

Then one day, my husband brought home a book for me by Dr. Joe Dispenza titled, "Breaking the Habit of Being Yourself." I felt like that was a nice hint from the husband that something about this process wasn't working, but I was too tired and sad to be offended so I cracked it open.

In addition to breaking down the physical nuances of our brains (something I found not only fascinating but actually really healing in a time where I had no idea what was going on with mine), Dr. Dispenza walks the reader through a step-by-step, full-body, guided meditation and how to achieve a higher state of being. Even typing this gives me the giggles because I just can't even believe I am sitting at my desk writing about meditation and a "higher state of being". This is my life now, I guess?

I went all-in on Dr. Dispenza's program. I read the book and downloaded the meditation sessions; I spent time everyday attempting to center myself and invoke visions of greatness and healing in my future. I studied and focused and did all that the book suggested.

How did it go? Well... Breaking the Habit is a fantastic resource with some awesome information and guidance within its cover. But I was a C-level student (at best) during this period of my life so a lot of the "focus" prompts were lost in my acute anxiety and, if I'm being truthful, my lack of sleep.

I was able to return to Dr. Dispenza's meditation routine over and over again and, with time, I did get better at practicing meditation. I don't know that I ever came out of C-level in his program but I did find moments of peace. And when moments are all that you are living for, they matter.

Meditation is a really difficult practice because of real life. Hard stop. Sometimes the hardest thing we can ask of ourselves to do is to take a minute to breathe. I am the mother to two littles and it seemed like every single time I sat down to try and center myself, someone needed a snack or their hair braided or a myriad of other things that are part of living. Life doesn't stop because of anxiety and that may have been one of the most difficult and sobering lessons for me to learn on my journey. So, if you are curious to find out how I take 40 minutes out of my day to center myself, here's the answer: I don't.

Meditation is called a practice for a reason: that is exactly what it takes. I began attempting to meditate fairly early on in my journey with panic and anxiety and it took over two months to even begin *feeling* it. There is this place you can come to in meditation where your mind is so focused that everything else kind of drifts away, at least that's the goal. I can recall exactly one time, early on in my practice, that the combination of exhaustion and attempted focus sent me into this state where I was fully aware of the nothingness around me but not fully present either; I felt like a total guru. Unfortunately, that was the first time and the last time it ever happened. Meditation in its textbook form continues to evade me to this day. It's something I attempt in the quiet minutes of a shower or driving, but generally speaking, my meditation practice has become my own – discarding the basic textbook tenants and trying to simply do whatever makes me feel centered.

After handfuls of weeks and twice as many visits to Dr. G, he politely let me know that I was on my own, I had graduated to the self-help section of my therapy program. Guys, this is a glaring sign of a good therapist and an amazing human being. Because therapy can stem from a really desperate place (panic attacks, for example), it is really easy for therapists to put us on the "forever plan" and continue to drag out our healing process (and our hourly rate) for a very long time. Dr. G and I were getting to a point where my visits were less frequent and starting to be filled with "let's review"-type conversations and I think in my gut, I knew it was time.

Dr. G told me his door was always open and reassured me that I would likely see him again and when that happened, it was nothing to be ashamed of. "Everyone needs a refresher from time-to-time," he said. I think that is true about most areas of our lives.

Here is the critical takeaway: Therapy didn't fix me. Therapy gave me the tools to help me fix myself, over and over again, for the rest of my life. Through a process of discovery and diagnosis and work, I was able to recognize the things in my life that were occupying more brain power and worry and angst than they should and address them. This is an amazing gift because that list of things won't always be the same, so being able to recognize those things as they appear and address them is truly the path to healing.

Therapy requires an expansive amount of trust. You have to trust your therapist and you have to trust the process. Most of the things Dr. G assigned me to do were on my "not for me" list just weeks before we met. But once I knew I trusted Dr. G, I had to let my guard down a bit and trust that what he had planned for me was far better than this rut I was in. I knew in my gut that Dr. G was the right therapist for me; like I said before, I was crazy lucky finding him on the first pull. But I'd like to think that if he wasn't the right one, I would have kept looking.

Therapy is a partnership, a gritty one. If you are considering therapy, don't force it. Trust your gut and know when you find a good partner to help guide you through whatever it is you are going through, you will know it.

The other half of that partnership is equally important: you. If your plan is to go into therapy as a skeptic, knowing it will never work, you are right. An assumption that you know everything will be the first indicator you will likely never get better. Plus, that seems like a giant contradiction to this gal so if you have that attitude, maybe skip it altogether. You have to be willing: willing to listen, willing to work, willing to change. None of these things are easy or comfortable or fun. But if you are willing, therapy might be a ticket to the peace you have been searching for.

Most importantly, let me save you some time and tell you to just ditch all of the pre-conceived notions you have about therapists and people who go to therapy and what that might do to your credibility. If there were truly a stigma, I've already thought of it and have been proven wrong.

When I first started talking with Dr. G, I was really nervous about what going to therapy said about me and my ability to function. I know he could tell that I was hesitant because in the middle of one early session, he said, "You aren't going to end up living under a bridge because of this." (Gosh, he's my hero.) He went on, "The people I see are some of the most put-together, successful, smart people around. They are organized and polite and rule-followers.

They try to be all the things… and that is why they are here." I hope that allows you to exhale, even just a little.

WORK

I've always tried to work hard, once I realized work would be the catalyst that led me to 'good' in life rather than simply 'good enough'. Work was a core value taught in my home growing up and we took it seriously enough that one of my cliché mantras, even to this day, is, "work hard, play hard." We are doing our best to teach our kids this same model, although most of the time, their rooms would scream otherwise.

Both of my parents worked full-time jobs while I was growing up, my mom as a civilian employee for the federal government and my dad a city employee in the state system. We went everywhere with our parents and saw firsthand the amount of work it took to run a household; we watched my mom run errands and helped her with the grocery shopping – I think every kid has memories of unloading the car in as few trips as possible (me, too) but my mom took the time to actually navigate the store with me, talking about price and needs versus wants. I learned a lot of valuable lessons about groceries and expenses on those trips. My brother spent a lot of time in the yard with my dad, mowing and washing vehicles and the like. I tried the riding lawn mower once growing up and our chain-link fence became a casualty of that war – so I stuck to grocery shopping and wiping down baseboards. (I have since learned my lesson and am an excellent mower now… with a push mower. I'm still nervous to attempt otherwise.) My point is that we helped – it was expected and we knew it.

My parents always made sure we looked nice – we got new clothes once in a while but mostly, they taught us how to take care of our things. My mom used to pay me 25 cents an item to iron our clothes which I thought was an amazing way to make money. Now I look back and realize how many hours she spent ironing everything we owned and I think she should have demanded a better allowance for herself. My parents gave us opportunities to learn and earn, both of which I am grateful for.

We didn't spend our entire lives working, although I'm sure at the time, we complained like we did. We had a ton of fun growing up; we took trips and started flying to exotic destinations (like Denver) when we were very young. We went boating and camping frequently, but never without at least a realization (I certainly could have been much more appreciative) of the work that went into making these things happen. We knew boating required gas money… and life jackets, and park entry fees as well as the dreaded expectation that we helped get ready to go and helped clean up when it was all over. Work was and is a way of life for my family.

As I got older, work continued to be a value I held onto with white knuckles. Whenever I encountered an issue, social or physical or mental, work was the way I ploughed through to the other side. If I stayed busy and worked hard enough, there were rarely issues I encountered that I couldn't get through and get through quickly. I felt this way about everything – school, work, family. Even in my perceived connection with God, work played a major role.

My relationship with God has always been amicable; I'd say there was a mutual understanding between the two of us that I would pray for things and then do all I could to force His hand into compliance with my plans. If I worked hard enough, I could make anything happen. I am now very aware that this is not how a normal relationship with any higher power is supposed to play out so please make a mental note that I recognize the error of my ways.

I don't know that I have ever consciously admitted to my exhausting pious perceptions until the last year, figuring that negotiating with God was likely this tough for everyone, but we just didn't speak of it. In my mind I guess I assumed everyone played a bit of a contradictory cat-and-mouse game when it came to asking and receiving guidance, help, advice or, if I worked hard enough, even miracles that have been granted to so many others. I figured the Bible stories were probably full of grunt work and back-and-forth, but who writes that stuff down? Nobody wants to read a piece-by-piece account of Noah testing the wood and chopping the wood and shaping the wood and failing and trying again when "building a boat" sums it up so nicely.

I tell you all of this not to simply talk about work but to lay a groundwork for how I initially decided to approach my anxiety; it shouldn't surprise you now that I told myself if I just worked hard enough, I could beat this and get back to my normal life.

At my first appointment with Dr. G, he had me push myself physically on an elliptical machine, right in the middle of a maniacal panic attack. (To be clear, this was very much related to MY specific issues and panic and would likely not be the advice your therapist would give you. Elliptical machines do not fix anxiety. I had a lot of issues about death that were nearly paralyzing me and Dr. G had a specific plan to help me move past them. Don't go run a mile during a panic attack unless your doctor tells you to, ok?) With the promise I would come out the other side in a better head space, Dr. G told me to go to work and run as hard as I could on that machine. So, I did. I ran harder and cried harder than I maybe have my entire life on that stupid machine. This was what I was waiting for – an instruction manual on how to feel better and if it required physical work, I was not shunning it.

I did feel a little calmer after my therapeutic cardio session, maybe from pure exhaustion, but a little better none-the-less. It didn't fix my issues long-term but what I did learn about myself in that moment was I was ready and willing to do whatever it would take to get better and I had just proven it by running in my ballet flats. In those few minutes, Dr. G physically pushed me to my limit; physical stress paired with mental turmoil is about as traumatic as I had experienced up to that point and I had two options to get out of it: push or quit. I wanted to heal. I wanted to be better. And this little exercise allowed me to see just how badly I wanted it. For several short minutes, I was able to overcome my mind and push myself past what I believed I was capable of handling. For the previous few days, I had nothing. No confidence, no hope, no future. But in those few minutes, I knew I had it in me to tackle this trial. I was ready. And I have held onto some portion of that confidence ever since.

Later in the process, Dr. G would joke that in that minute, he, too, knew I was ready to get to work and was serious about getting better. I was grateful he saw that in me because I don't know how hard he would have pushed me otherwise. I left his office that day with a laundry list of things I needed to start doing, more things I needed to stop doing, a follow-up appointment in just a few days and a glimmer of hope.

From the onset, I knew that work was *my* only way through this. Not only did a task list provide a nice distraction from my daily panic, it provided some much-needed order in a time of complete chaos. Because I couldn't make sense of my world, it became critical to set daily "goals" (you'll see how fluid this term can be once I get into their contents) that would provide some direction and normalcy, both to my life and the lives of my family. You have to remember that in the middle of all of this, I was a stay-at-home-mom with two kids (ages six and four) and a wife to a husband with a full-time job and a side hustle to boot. I also had a side business I was running and a nearly full-time volunteer position at my church. Life doesn't stop because you have anxiety so it was critical I did things (even small things) to make me and my people feel normal.

When I was first diagnosed, I felt like I had lost not only my sense of self but a sense of dignity that I felt I had carried my entire life; I was the strong one, the scheduler, the doer and finisher. I set goals and accomplished them, I set limits and never violated them. But with one subtle change, all of that was gone. I didn't know who I was nor who I would become when, if, this all resolved itself. I felt like a shell of a person I once was, wandering into the recesses of my mind to try and grasp a glimpse of the woman I was just the day before. I could remember her, but she was just outside of my reach.

At first, my goals were things like, "get dressed" or "shower" or "eat something". These are so rudimentary that they are almost painful to write; nobody wants to admit that they were in a dark enough place they had to be reminded to shower, but that's the reality of it. I spent several weeks trying to mentally latch onto anything that would get me out of bed; even a move downstairs to the couch could be considered a victory on some days and so I took it.

Little by little (as the showering became more regular), goals got a little more complex. I took Dr. G's advice to start writing things down and meditating. Some days (and I'm aware how contrary this is going to sound), even meditating and practicing gratitude were too overwhelming for me, so I didn't; in the midst of all of this, I had days where I said "no," even to therapy. And as the mighty Tabitha Brown says, "…and that's my business."

Saying "no" doesn't correlate well with being a workhorse… or so I thought. I was once told, "If you want something done, ask a busy person to do it. They are the ones getting things done." I took that, translated it, and internalized it to sound something like this: "If you want to be valuable to other people, stay busy. You aren't helpful if you say 'no'."

For those of you who have no issues managing your time as your own, that translation will likely make no sense and for that, I extend my congratulations. For those of you who struggle with owning your own time and using the word "no", you can totally sit by me.

As I've studied and grown through my anxiety and overcome my compulsive need to say "yes" to everything (apparently *that* is what gave me value?), I've learned a couple of critical things:

"No" and "Because I don't want to" are both perfectly good answers to give to a variety of questions. The end. You don't need to make up some story about your nephew's piano recital to get out of helping set up tables and you certainly don't need to fake an ulcer to get out of going on a walk with a neighbor. You saying "no" is a choice and when people ask you a question, you have the right to say it.

A couple of caveats about that previous paragraph: This is sound advice for adults or anyone who has built any sort of autonomy. If you are a teenager, living in your parent's basement and eating all their food, and your mom asks you to clean your room, "no" is not an acceptable choice, really. Nor is "no" a choice that allows you out of homework. Apply this "no" advice to time-sucks that won't inherently affect your future, mmmkay? And if I find out that anyone is using this advice irresponsibly or to put their mother in her place, I'm coming for you.

Also, this is not an excuse not to help. I stand behind the fact that serving other people made up some of the few times I felt remotely normal during all of this. Service is a great way to focus on others rather than dwell on your issues. I believe we should lend a hand wherever possible.

What I *am* saying is that you should be able to decide when to help, rather than having guilt dictate your actions. Guilt and anxiety are ugly stepsisters and having both nagging at you is awful. Guilt goes away when you decide to make deliberate choices with your time, for the right reasons.

Early in my therapy, Dr. G brought up the topic of self-care. He must have known my relationship with that term wasn't good because he immediately backed up to explain.

Many people interpret "self-care" as the ability to do whatever, whenever because "I am most important". I've seen many people (and relationships) destroyed by the selfish tendencies that come with such a flippant disregard for others; we simply cannot live this way.

What Dr. G proceeded to explain was that self-care isn't about getting weekly pedicures or shopping sprees (both things commonly associated with this topic), but about being deliberate with my time. If I chose to vacuum the living room one afternoon because I wanted to, that is self-care. Whereas vacuuming the living room because I am afraid of what my mother will think when she visits later is not self-care. Does that make sense?

Each of us is allotted 24 hours in a day and spending them at the beck and call of others will certainly lead to our demise. Be deliberate with your time. Say "no" to things that make you uncomfortable and things that won't lead to eventual growth. Guard your time as if it is sacred, because it is. The way you choose to spend your moments can have a drastic impact on both your happiness and your health. Find ways to spark joy in yourself and in others; if you spark it enough times, it will light a fire.

Battling through my anxiety diagnosis has been the most exhausting work I've ever done. But as I look back, it is probably some of the most rewarding. Any time you can expend your mental energy and your physical strength on something you know will make you a better person, the gratification is inescapable. Satisfaction with that work isn't always immediate, but the work and those feelings come hand-in-hand and cannot be separated. Being intentional with your time and your "yes" are critical components to healing from any sort of mental anguish. And the work is worth it.

MEDICAL HELP

Medical intervention was the second path I trudged after my panic started (the third if you count self-loathing and 'ignoring it' as a step, I guess), two days after my first visit to a licensed therapist. But I want to be clear that I didn't initially schedule the appointment to deal with my anxiety; I scheduled the appointment to deal with some really uncomfortable symptoms I was feeling – I thought I was getting the flu.

I woke up one morning in December 2018 feeling rummy; my head ached and my muscles were sore from my shoulders to my feet. I remember circling the couch, sitting and rising every few minutes in prayer that the elevation change would do something to clear my head. Things got progressively worse as the morning went on and my head just didn't feel right. In addition, my heart was racing and my stomach had seen better days.

Having two little kids to care for at the time, I started to worry about whether or not I'd be able to stay on my feet long enough to help them when they needed it throughout the day. So, I did what all grown women long to do in times like these: I called my mom. My mom has always been such a support to me and my family, regardless of the situation or demands on her and her time, and my dive into the deep end of anxiety was no different. She and my dad were overwhelmingly generous with their time and resources during my healing process and aside from recommending that I see a therapist, this day was the real start of their journey with me and anxiety.

We arrived at the doctor's office and I told the receptionist I needed to be seen for anxiety and panic attacks. This had not been the discussion nor the feeling all morning, I just assumed I was getting sick. Because I had never known panic previously nor physical affects from anxiety, being able to know this was the issue that needed addressing was as foreign to me as picking my favorite oyster. It is a miracle that those self-diagnostic words came out of my mouth as they certainly weren't mine but were exactly what I needed to say at that moment.

I remember going on my first visit to Snow College during my senior year in high school and sitting down with an academic advisor to discuss what Snow had to offer. After a few minutes of chatter, the advisor asked me what my major was going to be. I was very academic in high school, I studied hard and I was involved in a lot of different programs. But because of that, I didn't really have any clear direction on what I wanted to be when I grew up. I had tossed around law school and education, potentially business, but I certainly hadn't made up my mind as to my college major. But, without hesitation, I looked at the advisor and said, "Communications. That is my major." And then I proceeded to sit there with my mouth agape, initially wondering where that came from and then being mortified because I didn't even know if 'communications' *was* a major. Did I just tell this advisor I wanted to major in talking? Great start, Car. Get that college degree.

You can imagine my surprise when the advisor smiled and said, "I think you would be a great fit." We proceeded to talk about all of the opportunities for Comm majors at Snow, opportunities that would become an integral part of my education over the next two years, and I just felt it. This was not only the right school for me but something, somewhere had guided me to my most perfect educational path as a Communications major at a small junior college in Central Utah. That slip-of-the-tongue afforded me opportunities to write for and edit the school newspaper, work at the radio station, and meet some of the greatest people I know.

I believe there are moments in our lives, moments that matter and will direct the course of our history for years to come, where God has no choice but to step in and take us by the hand and physically set us on the right path. I very much believe in agency and that our ability to choose our destiny is a God-given right we've each been blessed with. But I also believe that God's love for each of us supersedes even the best explanations and that while He spends most of our lives gently nudging us in the right direction, occasionally, He must grab us by the shoulders and turn.

That morning when I told the clinic receptionist why I was there, I surprised myself but I knew in that minute it was right – I was there because of my anxiety. Every part of me knew it and I literally felt my shoulders turn toward the path that was inevitably mine.

My regular doctor (who I adore and will talk about in more detail) wasn't available that day so I met with a different family practitioner to discuss my issues. The minute he walked in the door and asked what he could do for me, I broke. I started weeping, uncontrollably, for what seemed like forever but likely was only a minute. When I couldn't get the words out, my mom stepped in and asked the doctor for anxiety medication. In that second, I felt like I was five years old. I was a kid all over again, feeling sick, and needing my mom so very much. I was terrified of what the doctor would say and I knew that whatever was currently happening to my mind and body was just the beginning. I was officially sick.

Once I was able to calm down a bit, I talked to the doctor about the previous couple of weeks, my panic attacks, my inability to sleep and the symptoms I had been experiencing that very morning. He asked me if there was anything I thought could be making me sick or worried right now and as noted earlier, I told him that I was supposed to have another therapy appointment that afternoon. He immediately nodded and slowed his questioning down.

The doctor proceeded to tell me that based on what we had discussed, it appeared as though my panic attacks weren't a few isolated incidents but that they were likely continuing to happen, over and over again. In fact, he said, I had likely experienced a panic attack in my sleep the previous night and that was what led to the headache, sore muscles and general feelings of uneasiness.

I had a lot of "ah-ha" moments through this process, many of them in those first few weeks and the mention of sleep-panic was one of those moments; not only did I have no idea our bodies were capable of such a nightmare, but I realized I had completely lost control of mine.

Growing up, I had gotten injured playing sports but never encountered anything that didn't mend quickly. I had gotten plenty of sprains but never a broken bone. When I was in my first years as a business professional, I took a softball to the face during a corporate softball game; it caused my forehead to swell, my eyes to turn black, and a really, really great homecoming at work the following day, but I got over it. With the exception of some scar tissue over my eyebrow that gets really red when it's hot (you can't make this stuff up), I had been fairly injury-free for 36 years. So, when I realized my mind and my body were embarking on a pretty sadistic journey together, I wasn't sure how to respond.

The doctor recommended I start on a mild dose of Klonopin, a medication used to treat panic disorders and hopefully, take the edge off enough to let me sleep. He also initially recommended I take Xanex when needed. Xanex is also used to treat anxiety, but is a much faster release so it enters your blood stream much quicker and provides relief in the event of the sudden onset of a panic attack. Lastly, he gave me some nausea medication. Ever since I had my sweet babes, my stomach has been, how you say, not so good. But the anxiety had taken it to a whole new level and it had been several days since I was able to keep anything down. Dehydration was starting to set in and the doctor emphasized our need to get it under control.

I know how crazy all of this sounds to anyone reading it, potentially even those who have experienced anxiety but suffered different side-effects. Even I think I sound like a professional hypochondriac when I start listing all of the things my body was doing at the time, from dehydration to muscle weakness and headaches; I guess it should be no wonder that I was 100% sure I was going to die.

The physical side-effects of anxiety are an interesting study all by themselves. When your adrenaline kicks in, your internal systems go into hyperdrive, trying to make sense of your environment. Many people who struggle with anxiety and depression also struggle with a host of physical ailments that are brought on by their emotional battles; headaches, muscle tension and soreness, abdominal pain, indigestion, dizziness, sight-issues, migraines, and lethargy can all be side-effects of anxiety, along with a myriad of other issues. The hardest part is that while the physical ailments aren't real (your stomach isn't really melting lava inside of you), they *feel* real.

This disparity can lead to a LOT of frustration when anxiety-sufferers visit medical doctors with what feel like serious ailments only to be given a clean bill of health. I know I'm likely pointing out the obvious… but this leads to further anxiety, wondering if the doctor possibly missed something or, on a simpler but no-less-true note, that now your file contains a memo about you being either a) crazy or b) a hypochondriac.

I remember shortly after I was put on Xanex (within 24 hours), I ended up in the emergency room in the wee hours of the morning. I had never really taken pills beyond over-the-counter medications and acid reducers so I wasn't prepared for the changes a pill like this would have on my body. Xanex made me feel, well, not great.*
Shortly after taking my prescribed dose, I starting feeling jittery and

nervous. Because I hadn't been able to keep any food or water down that day because of my stomach issues, things took a quick turn for the worse. Half way through the night, I started feeling like by body was thawing, like that feeling after coming in from the snow and taking a warm bath, but this thaw was happening in my abdomen and chest and it was terrifying.

After a long night of pacing in and out and around my old room at my parents' home, we made our way to the emergency room at our local hospital and I started getting fluids for some mild dehydration and the staff started to run basic blood pressure and heart rate tests. After speaking with the doctor, he decided to run a full blood panel to ensure everything was normal. As we waited for the results, I sat in the hospital bed and just hoped they would find something wrong. All I wanted was an answer – if they could find something in my bloodwork that could explain away the pain and the panic, we could fix it and I could go back to my regularly scheduled programming.

It shouldn't be any surprise at this point in the story that my bloodwork came back completely regular. If it hadn't, I would have gotten treatment for whatever was ailing my poor body and it would all be a distant memory. Instead, as the emergency room doctor sat with me and told me my bloodwork was normal, I remember looking him in the face and saying, "Now you think I'm crazy, right? I'm feeling so terrible and something is definitely wrong and all the tests say I should be fine and now I have to face the fact that I may be crazy and you are looking at me like I'm making this all up."

To be fair, while the doctor didn't have the best bedside manner, he certainly wasn't looking at me like I was crazy. In fact, he was completely methodical in his delivery and in telling me that I was just going to have to ride out the medications I was on until I got feeling better. I am super grateful that I did push a little bit though because he put me on a much, much better nausea medication and pumped me full of fluids while I was there so when I walked out, I didn't feel like it was a total waste of money… I mean "time".

I think there is a lesson in all of this, one I've thought through over and over again. When I was in the beginning of this process, I didn't know what was happening to me or how to fix it or where to turn. I, more than anyone, recognized my thoughts weren't normal – but that didn't keep me from thinking them. I was scared. And I think more than anything, I needed someone to say, "I believe you and everything is going to be alright." It was some time before I heard anything like that from anyone, not because they weren't willing to say it but because this thing, this trial, was new to them, too.

I think when we see someone in our lives suffering, it is easy to throw sympathy around and then go about our normal business. We extend condolences when someone dies, we drop off a card when a dog goes missing; our intentions are always good and I think doing small, caring acts is a million times better than doing nothing. Edmund Burke once said, "Nobody made a greater mistake than he who did nothing because he could do only a little." I believe that enough to have it hanging in my kitchen, so please don't misunderstand my intent.

What I do wonder is at what point do people have to suffer for us to change our tune from, "I'm sorry that happened. I'm sure it's hard," to, "I'm sorry that happened and I'll be sitting here, holding your hand, until you ask me to stop." How bad do things have to be for us to really honor our covenant to mourn with those that mourn? I'm certainly guilty of dropping off a meal and then dropping off the face of someone's Earth mere minutes later. My follow-through stinks, even to this day. But I remember those first few weeks of really being sick and the things that meant the most to me: it was my mom having my bed ready when I got home from the hospital that morning and not even asking what she could do for my kids, but just doing it, like always, without questions; it was my husband sitting with me through that first night at my parent's house, watching me convulse and shiver and cry and not saying anything, just sitting with me and encouraging me to drink; it was my forever-intuitive friend showing up with an extremely large soda one afternoon and, while I was grateful for the soda, I was most grateful when she just let me cry in the driveway. The list goes on to include a best friend sitting in my living room and laugh-crying with me about how stupid life can be at times, and my brother reminding me that, "...God hath not given us the spirit of fear; but of power, and of love, and of a sound mind," (2 Timothy 1:7, KJV). The list goes on to include dozens of other seemingly insignificant acts by people who let me know they were *my* people, that no matter what was to come my way (and it would be a lot) they were not just cheering me on but would be there to go through it, hand-in-hand, right by my side.

This kind of compassion goes beyond the textbook condolences we've been trained to give. I think each of us has a compassion standard we are "good" at – something we do frequently to show our contribution without making ourselves uncomfortable. For some people it is hand-written notes, for others it is a text message. My compassion default is food; if someone's family member dies, I drop off food. If they are having a bad week, I bring food. If we are celebrating something? You guessed it, food. Food is easy and not just because we all love it and need it, making it difficult to turn down or read too much into. Food is easy for me because it becomes my complete offering and allows me to hide behind it, not exposing the tender parts of me to the recipient. Because of food, I don't have to sit in silence, with me as the sole offering, in a living room filled with grief. Food allows me to congratulate someone else's accomplishments quickly and then get in my car and wonder when it will be my turn to waltz with success. Food is my indicator that, "I see you and care about what is going on with you, but I'm going to do it from the porch."

I think soul-stretching compassion can be such a gift, both to us and the recipient. Sometimes our best offering is us, stripped free of cards and lasagnas and articles on how to feel better. Other times, our very best offering *is* a card or a lasagna or an article on how to feel better… when it comes from the tender reaches of your soul and not from a sense of guilt or obligation. One thing I have learned through all of this is that regardless of your compassion channel of choice, the intent always, *always* comes through.

Not long after my emergency room run-in, I set an appointment so see my regular primary-care physician to discuss a longer-term plan for recovery and regular monitoring of my situation. It had been a couple of weeks since I had been in the hospital and I was ready to take medications that would help to fix this mess rather than make me feel numb to all of it.

Spoiler alert: my primary-care physician ends up being another hero in this story. I've become a major advocate for this relationship and hope you are in a position to have someone who knows your health history and is constantly looking out for your best interest. I know this isn't the case for everyone and some see it as unnecessary but, as you can see from my story, you just never know.

I walked into Dr. S's office a shell of my former self, both physically and mentally. In the previous four weeks, I had dropped nearly 25 pounds (before you ask, no. I would not recommend this diet.) and I felt and looked hollow. I'm pretty sure I was in sweats and cried virtually the entire time.

Dr. S knew me from years of annual visits and could tell this wasn't normal. As I talked with him about the previous three weeks, he did what so many doctors struggle to do – he listened. Intently. And with the sympathy I thought I could only garner from my mother. It wasn't condescending or smug; it was completely sincere in a way that made me feel totally safe. I can still picture those moments in my minds' eye and can literally feel how it felt to be heard, really heard, for the first time in several agonizing weeks. It has been more than two years since that interaction and I still can't think about it without gratitude coming out of my eyes.

Thankfully, Dr. S was full of wisdom. Not only was I not his first patient with anxiety (you'd be hard-pressed to find a doctor with no experience), but he was ready and willing to help me slowly work through all of this until I was whole.

I feel like it has been a couple of pages so it seems like a good time to remind you that none of this is medical advice for you or anyone you may know. As I talk through *my* specific diagnosis and subsequent prescriptions, please note it is for recollection purposes and not diagnostic ones. Please don't march into your PCP and demand similar medications or treatments and extra please don't try to buy some on the street. Take this for what it is: a glimmer of hope that there *are* answers. But they will likely be different for each of us.

After some discussion about my feelings on Klonopin and Xanex, Dr. S recommended I start on a low dose of an SSRI called Lexapro. Selective Serotonin Reuptake Inhibitors (SSRI) work to restore balance of the serotonin levels in your brain by blocking the reuptake of serotonin by neurons, increasing its availability in the brain, hopefully increasing mood. Basically, they make your body use less serotonin and pump extra to your brain. SSRIs are a different class of medication than some anti-depressants and after some discussion, this felt like a good starting place for me. Dr. S and I discussed potential side-effects and dosing (mine would be fairly low) and in a moment that I didn't see coming, he dropped the bomb:

"You should start feeling a little better in four to six weeks. You should really start feeling better in eight weeks, but it can take some people as long as 12."

Eight weeks? Not tomorrow? I know that sounds demanding but after a couple of weeks of little-to-no sleep and absolute emotional turmoil, eight weeks is nearly a death sentence. On top of that, there was no guarantee Lexapro would be my answer. Everybody's system responds differently to medication and there was a good chance I would take Lexapro for weeks, feel nothing, and need to start the process over with a totally different medication. I politely told Dr. S that I felt like asking me to do that was like staring down the barrel of a gun. To which he replied, "I know."

Please know I don't make those statements lightly nor in jest. Please let me be very clear about something in this moment – the road to healing anxiety, regardless of the method you choose or the help you seek, is not a short one. It is long and bumpy and arduous. The hard part is that every minute of panic feels like an hour so you can imagine what an eight-week outlook (with a potential do-over) feels like. So many people wait so long to seek help that eight weeks isn't just difficult, it is impossible, and they find themselves looking to more drastic substances or actions for relief. Please, hear my pleading: don't wait to talk to someone. Don't wait until it is too hard. There are resources available that *will* make you better, but it is trial and error and the sooner you start, whether it be with a doctor or a therapist, the better off you will be.

Dr. S and I agreed I would hang on to the Xanex for emergencies, all-the-while knowing I'd never take it again. And we agreed to touch base in a few weeks.

Like all of the other parts of this journey, my relationship with Lexapro was a process; can't something just *once* go off without a hitch?! I remember sitting in church about a week after I began taking the medication and feeling a little dizzy. As I looked up from my "don't talk to me" posture, I felt my head move into some sort of draining process. It started at the top of my forehead and slowly worked its way down to my temples and past my eyes. It didn't hurt, but it certainly wasn't normal. I felt like the frontal lobe of my brain was coming alive and as I sat there, I was quietly preparing myself for a return trip to the hospital. I was also starting to wonder if they offered punch cards for frequent visitors, hoping that maybe enough of these visits would at least score me a free blood draw.

After a few minutes, the feelings subsided and I was left with a monster headache. That brain-drain feeling never returned and it was chalked up to the medication possibly opening up some capillaries and essentially breathing life into parts of my brain for the first time in a long time.

It's weird to draw these parallels as I look back now but that was such a key one for me, the breathing life into me for the first time in a long while. Sometimes, we don't know the kind of mental shape we are in until we are forced to make a change. I spent years simply surviving on "good enough", never knowing how different and how much better I could feel. It took some drastic changes (and pretty major breakdowns) for me to realize exactly how bad it had gotten and how desperately I needed help.

I am continually grateful for a doctor who took the time to get me through a lengthy trial process with Lexapro. Over the next four weeks, I saw some incremental improvement in how I was feeling – I certainly cried less. I experienced minimal side-effects on my medication and started to feel functional again. It took another eight weeks to really feel like a steady version of myself and to settle into taking Lexapro daily. That's 12 weeks for those of you counting.

When Dr. S and I originally spoke, he told me I would be on medication for at least six months (potentially longer) and I would have to work up to my allotted dosage as well as ween off the medication if the opportunity presented itself down the road; while it wasn't habit forming, SSRIs are not something to stop taking cold-turkey. So, once I worked up to my full dose and was feeling somewhat better, I did the practical thing and started counting down the days until I would be medication-free; *obviously* I was a strong woman who just needed some temporary help and these pills, in conjunction with the hard work I was doing in therapy, would heal me in those six months.

Obviously.

*It's important to note that everyone reacts differently to medication. For some, properly prescribed anxiety medication like Xanex can be a life-changer, producing calming effects that allow for proper perspective. For me, this was not the case. It is so very important to consult with a trained medical professional before attempting any type of medication for panic disorders and anxiety. It is equally important to speak up when they don't feel good. Finding the right medication and the right dosing can be a fairly tricky game but it is one I know a good doctor will work with you on, should medication be necessary.

A LONG DECEMBER

Every year, my husband and I have a standing date night on December 23rd. We used to go out to dinner and stay in a nice hotel and just enjoy the day before everything got crazy with family obligations and dinners and the like. As our marriage has progressed and kids have taken over, some of our date nights consist of takeout and a quiet night at home while our kids stay with their grandparents. Either way, it is a win for us and for the kids as we all spend some much-needed time apart before the sugar and gift marathon begins.

In 2018, I was a couple of weeks into my battle with panic and anxiety when our annual date-night surfaced. Trevor had been in charge of planning it this year and had scheduled an outing for us up Logan Canyon, a winter haven for outdoor enthusiasts who didn't mind the cold. So much had happened between Trevor initially booking our trip and us actually going, I wasn't really sure how to react when he told me he had rented snowmobiles for a full day of frolicking in the snow and then a relaxing night at a lodge just over the ridge from Bear Lake, my favorite place in the world.

There are a few things I need to pause and tell you before we go any further. First, I don't like the snow. Really at all. I don't like being cold and would absolutely never survive a night in an igloo. So, my trepidation about this outing was already high, recent diagnosis excluded. Trevor reassured me that once we got moving on the sleds, I wouldn't really notice the cold. Plus, he took extra precautions by securing me some toasty new gloves and a pair of snow pants that were every fashion blogger's dream.

Second, I am not an experienced snowmobiler. I have ridden multiple four-wheelers and wave runners throughout my life but a snowmobile was not in my repertoire. I was completely unprepared for the physical work it takes to maneuver one of these machines through the backwoods. I assumed we would find a nicely-groomed trail somewhere and cruise the day away, spotting rabbits and families of deer, just like a cartoon dream.

For those of you wondering: yes, I should have said "no thanks" to this endeavor, based solely on my anxiety. I know that now. But when you have been crying for two weeks and feeling guilty for sending your "normal" family life into a tailspin, you do crazy things to avoid wrecking yet another weekend plan. Plus, the idea of sitting alone in a hotel room while my husband was on the side of a snow-filled mountain didn't exactly calm my anxiety, so I went for it. At least we would be together.

That morning at breakfast and before the day's adventures, I took a Xanex to help ease my nerves. This was not the wisest move I have ever made. Hard stop. Pills mixed with heavy machinery is a dangerous recipe, I know that. I can't recall if it actually issued that warning on the label, but let's assume it did and call this move of mine "totally idiotic". But I make this point because my previous rule-following-self would have never done this. If nothing else, this should (again) illustrate how desperate I was to get back to normal; I didn't want to spoil the plans, I didn't want to sit alone. I just wanted to do what I would have always done and every time I took one of those pills, I washed it down with an eternal hope that this would be the one that "fixed" things.

We arrived at the mountain and as we were preparing to go on a "go at your own pace" ride, the manager of the snowmobiles told us they had some extra room in a guided tour that was heading out for the day if we wanted to jump in the group. This moment was pivotal for how the day would turn out. The logical side of me thought about how much safer it would be to go out with a guide and have someone with us in case our amateur ways got us into trouble. Trevor felt the same thing and signed us up for the group tour.

What didn't cross my mind is that following an experienced twenty-something into the backwoods of Logan canyon would pose its own issues; we were about to follow some snow cowboys into much rougher terrain than we would ever tackle ourselves... and we were about to do it for eight hours.

We set off on our adventure and for the first 20 or so minutes, we crossed open spaces and fairly flat terrain that allowed me to think and center myself. I figured if this were the kind of ride we would be in for, I could certainly spend the day with my thoughts, feeling safe in my skin. Things took a quick turn once we approached a line of trees, just up a short hill.

The snow and the terrain shifted from smooth to thick powder in a matter of feet. For those of you who are inexperienced with snowmobiling (as I most certainly was), this can cause a few issues, not the least of which being a sinking sensation and a strict demand to keep your weight evenly distributed, balanced and pushed forward. If you slow your machine down in these conditions (which a new snowmobile operator tends to do, frequently), you get one thing: stuck. I was stuck. And holding up our group of riders – the inconvenience I never like to be and immediately sparks my anxiety pilot light. My machine stalled and I slowly rolled off the side and into a snowbank. Flustered, I tried to quickly recover and found myself resembling Randy in "A Christmas Story", rolling around in the snow, unable to get up. More pressure, more anxiety.

As I got back to my machine and looked forward, I realized I had no idea what I had gotten myself into. The trees up ahead staggered themselves on the hillside, forming a tight maze for skilled adventurers to work through. The only problem was that I was *not* a skilled adventurer. I was prepared to ride around open spaces and frolic in the snow; I was not prepared for this.

Once our guide helped me (read: drove my machine) through this initial pass, I was determined to not spend the rest of the day looking like a total idiot. I'm sure I wasn't the worst driver they had ever seen, but in my anxiety-ridden state, I certainly was. My heart rate had escalated and my breathing had quickened and I was setting off on an eight-hour adventure on the cusp of another panic attack.

Winter sports especially take everything out of you, mentally and physically. Dealing with mother nature and her icy tricks can be dangerous so for this worried mess, I was on high alert for branches and sink holes and rough terrain. I held on to my machine with a vice grip that the jaws of life would have thought twice about attempting to loosen. My muscles were in a state of tension for the entire ride that day, making the repeated tumbles I took off of my machine that much more arduous.

As we drove, I found myself crying. I was scared and tired and staring down seven and a half additional hours of this little adventure. Between my sobs, I could hear my deep, panicked breathing under my helmet and the cloth face shield that had been given to me to keep me warm. I knew in my mind that the only way out of this was to go forward, there was no turning back to the safety and warmth of the lodge. My only way out was through the woods and the terrain and the ice and all the things I was terrified of.

We continued to ride (and sob) through the trees until we finally came to this wide-open bowl in the middle of the woods. There were feet of fresh, un-ridden snow and it was glittery and beautiful. Our guide told us this was a stopping point and that we could ride around for a little while and "play". Trevor checked in to make sure I was ok and then went off to ride over acres of fresh powder and I sat at the edge of the bowl, watching him and breathing and crying. When the other riders in our group were in the distance, I heard a muffled sound that barely sounded like words. "You're ok. You're ok. It's ok. You're ok." I was repeating this to myself, over and over again, without even realizing the words were actually coming out of my own mouth. I still wonder how long those words were actually coming out and not just living in my head that day.

I removed my helmet and my face shield and let the cold air hit my face. As I sat and looked at the bowl of snow below me, I started to talk. I don't know that at the time I would have qualified my rantings as a 'prayer', but now that I look back, I certainly would. I needed to know that what I was saying to myself was true – "Am I really ok? Is everything really going to be ok? Am I going to get through today and tomorrow and next week? I'm destroyed and alone and tired. How am I going to be ok?"

Minutes later, Trevor and I met up again and as we spoke, he realized that somewhere, in this wide-open plot of freshly laid snowmobile tracks that covered as far as the eye could see, he had lost his cell phone. Is it the world's biggest tragedy? No. Did it feel like it at the moment? Yes. One minute you are pouring your angsty heart out to God about your survival and the next moment, you are looking at acres and acres of snow, knowing that there was no way to recover what was lost. I was devastated and angry that this stupid day had cost me my sanity and my energy and now an expensive phone I didn't know how we were going to replace.

But, in a habitual moment of normalcy, we did what we always do: Trevor said a quick prayer and went to work. We took off on our machines and started crisscrossing the acres of open land he had been riding. We went up hills and in trees. I fell off a couple of times and sat and sulked, but got back up and kept riding. About 15 minutes into our search, just as I had given up, I saw Trevor, standing in the center of the bowl, waving his arm with a cold but still working phone in his hand. I was stunned.

It is interesting now, several years later, to look back and realize what a parallel that day ran to my everyday life at the time. Heading into my battle with anxiety felt just like entering those woods. The course I was about to embark on was clearly beyond my level of expertise, and when I fell and couldn't make it, it was embarrassing and frustrating and exhausting. I needed the help of our guide to navigate the rough parts. Don't get me wrong – I very much wanted to navigate the trail on my own but there were just areas that weren't possible to make it through as an amateur rider. It was especially humiliating when everyone else seemed to be navigating the terrain with apparent ease and I just couldn't do it.

Anxiety can feel like that – like you are trying to figure out how to carry five bowling balls with your bare hands, and everyone around you seems to have been given a cart with wheels. It feels like you signed up for the advanced life course on a beginner's skill level. It is intimidating and uncomfortable and can leave you looking behind you, wishing to go back to the safety of when things were easy and comfortable.

The problem with looking back is that the only way to do it safely is to stop moving, and what good does that do you? I knew the only way out of those woods that day was simply to move forward. I wasn't going to like it, I didn't even know how I would make it or how long it would last, but I knew I had to do it. Staying still wasn't an option; the only thing I wanted less than the ride that day was sitting in the cold, waiting to be rescued. I was *not* going down like that. If I were going to be rescued, it would be in the midst of a brutal fight with that mountain.

In the moment that Trevor told me he had lost his cell phone, I almost broke. It was so dumb but it was that "one more thing" I just couldn't process at the time. I didn't know what to do. There was a two percent chance we would find that phone, buried in the feet of powder and tracks that he had been riding in. It just wasn't possible for us to find it. But God knew better.

As we prayed for help that afternoon, I distinctly remember wondering if we should sit quiet and hope someone would call his phone. This approach would have been a genius way for God to answer our prayers, but even He couldn't get cell service in those woods. So, when that plan scratched, our only option was to do work. The odds were slim but that didn't mean we couldn't try. So, try we did.

Sometimes, navigating mental health can feel like a futile search through the snow. There is no real beginning or rule book as to where to start making sense of it all. And in fact, if you just sit back on the edge and look at all that is in front of you to sift through, it can be daunting to the point of giving up. Please don't give up. Despite the tracks and the mud and the impossible-ness of it all, simply trying is the right place to start.

When Trev finally found his phone, I felt such relief for about two minutes. For two minutes I felt loved and heard and felt like my prayers were actually answered. And then sadness sank back in because #anxiety. But for those two minutes, I was distracted and amazed and grateful. And it felt good.

My anxiety perspective has continued this same dance to this day: back-and-forth with God in what feels like endless negotiations for even the smallest sign that He is there. He lets me struggle for a while, hoping I will put in the work and learn as I go. Then, out of seemingly nowhere, He appears. When we found the phone, it had nothing to do with my initial pleading to help me know I would be ok. But it was *something*, a miracle to remind me they still exist. And while He didn't take away my sadness or my fear, it was enough to bring me hope that one day, if I keep sifting, I will find my miracle as well.

STIGMA

When I first went on anxiety medication, I could barely handle the fact that it would take me at least six weeks to even start seeing its benefit. As I've said, two months seems impossible when every day seems like a thousand. But the minute I did start feeling better, I did what a lot of anxiety suffers do: I started checking the calendar and waiting for the day I could start transitioning off my meds. Sounds ambitious, right?

There is a stigma that comes with taking medications for psychotic ailments, one that is depicted in movie after movie where a patient in a fluffy robe is issued their daily pills in a little plastic cup. I never consciously paid attention to that stigma really, and why would I? I would never need medications to help control my brain function or my emotional state.

When I was finally diagnosed and prescribed an SSRI, my first and only thought was how I would keep it quiet until I could transition off. My family knew what was going on but they had to love me, "crazy" or not. I had a boiling worry that my neighbors or other friends would find out I was taking pills and I'd quickly inherit the title of "neighborhood psycho", a judgment on them that certainly was not fair, nor ever came to fruition.

Even without the social pressure of being different, I'm going to say what any anxiety, OCD, depression sufferer has thought at some point or another: I didn't want to be the crazy lady. Call it a misconception on my part or an irrational categorization on the part of society, those pills come with a healthy dose of humility and a want to quietly disappear into the fray.

So, as soon as I started feeling better, I made a plan to work with my doctor to transition off the pills as soon as the allotted six months of minimum treatment were up; I'd be free by July and back to my spunky self in no time.

It's horribly unnecessary to paint a picture of the irony in all of this; even as I type, I see the error of my ways. I was feeling better in part *because* of the medication, not because I was magically cured of the misfiring in my brain. I took my signs of wellness as the pre-school sign of being "all better" when in fact, I was still in the very, very early stages of my battle with anxiety.

I have since learned this is a fairly common reaction amongst those who are initially prescribed medication for psychotic episodes. That stigma, the one that often accompanies taking these medications, causes a lot of patients to feel shame or embarrassment. So, in hopes of alleviating that shame, they quit taking their medications in their early stages of treatment, assuming their problem is "solved" because they are starting to feel better. Patients justify this by telling themselves that this must have just been an isolated incident and medication was probably an overkill, or that their problem is something that will eventually just "go away" if they will just push through and figure out how to not worry so much. This mentality is both physically dangerous and mentally harmful; not only is an abrupt end to these medications physically shocking to your body and puts your already fragile mental and emotional state at risk, I can unequivocally say that no amount of "happy" or good news or "cheering up" will alleviate an actual chemical misnomer in your brain. It just won't.

When I eventually relapsed, (spoiler alert: I relapsed) my perception of being on medication was the unspoken elephant in the room. Dr.

S. calmly looked at me, with all the sympathy I'm sure he could muster, and said, "I think we should plan on this being a part of your regimen for the foreseeable future." I can only imagine my disappointment was strewn across my face because he followed up with, "You know, Carlee, if you were in here because you had a blood disorder or diabetes or issues with your liver, we'd give you medication and nobody would even think twice about it because it is what you needed to function normally. In fact, you would likely be so grateful you were able to find help. You need to be ok with the fact that it is the same thing we are doing *for your brain*. There is nothing to be done about this except giving your brain the added support it needs to process life like it should." Not once did he use the word "crazy". And that felt good.

It took me over a year of being on medication to be 'ok' with it. The funny part is, over that time and frankly, never in my life, has anyone approached me to ask me what pills I take in the morning, let alone what they are for. What was I so afraid of? My doctor finding out I take anxiety medication when his signature was on the prescription? Who did I have to answer to about my illness and why was I so embarrassed I needed help?

I think the big worry stemmed from the fact that I was battling an invisible monster. Anxiety fighters are warriors, sent into battle on a hope and a prayer, to fight a demon that only exists in the recesses of their mind. When a person breaks their leg, it is obvious to those around them they are in need of some added grace; nobody would (or should) tell a person on crutches to hurry up. I wish the same patience existed for those struggling with mental disorders but unfortunately, there is no way to know what is happening inside someone's mind until they are willing to disclose it. My husband and I joke that I should start a t-shirt line for invisible medical diagnoses; mine would say, "Clinically, I want it more." That might stimulate more patience for those of us struggling.

Or maybe the answer is to just treat everyone like they are struggling with something we can't see. I don't think we need to go around with kid gloves on 24 hours a day, but maybe a little added patience with and care for those around us wouldn't be such a harmful thing. I can almost guarantee that more than a handful of people who know me WELL are going to be stunned by what I've revealed in these chapters; many of them have no idea I ever had anxiety issues, nor that I continue to deal with them even today. I often wonder how many others are sitting near me, stuck in their own quiet battles with physical or mental or spiritual health, afraid or unwilling or even unable to discuss them, silently pleading for someone to extend any added amount of grace.

Maybe if we just assumed everyone was a mosaic, made up of cracks and mis-colored pieces, fighting to stay together and appear whole, we could be more tender, more sympathetic, more patient. We might end up being the glue that holds them together, even for another minute, and keeps it from shattering into a thousand distorted pieces.

SACRED THINGS

In addition to therapy and medical intervention, I sought help and advice from wherever I could get it. People are generally well-intentioned, especially when it comes to dealing out wisdom on how to fix the problems we are having in our lives. I've found this particularly true of religious folks; there is certainly no shortage of encouragement to pray away the bad in your life with a quick follow-up promise that prayer will fix things… or at a very minimum, make you feel better. I was encouraged dozens of times (again, all by well-intentioned people) to "pray away" my anxiety and God would certainly make me feel better. But here was my problem:

I couldn't pray. Not like I used to.

I always relied on formal prayer to guide me through whatever rough patches I was experiencing in my life – I would have troubles and I would pray to God for answers or guidance or miracles I knew only He could provide. Now, in my darkest hours, my *only* communication with the heavens came in the form of desperate pleading for just a moment of relief from the sadness and worry; there was nothing formal about it – no addressing God as the majesty I've always known Him to be but just dire crying out for mercy that seemed no closer than it did in the previous night's appeals.

The part that was most difficult for me during all of this was the sense I was totally and completely alone in my struggle; culturally, we are taught that help is always a simple prayer away and if we will just pray with full purpose of heart, we will be filled with the gift of the Spirit

– The Comforter – that will ease our minds and our hearts and bring peace.

I can recall the first several weeks after my initial diagnosis and the nights I stayed awake, crying on my bed and begging for relief. The guttural moans coming from deep in me are what my nightmares are now made of; I can still see myself, curled on my bed, wailing and begging for someone to make the pain go away. I had physical discomfort, yes, but the sorrow I felt in my head and in my heart was unbearable. I was more than fractured – I was broken.

People wonder all the time if their prayers are reaching the heavens; I knew mine weren't. This time was different though than other times I had struggled to commune with God. I didn't just feel like my prayers were bouncing off some invisible ceiling and making their way back to my heart. This time, it felt like my prayers hit that ceiling and shattered into a million pieces, scattering at my feet in unrecognizable shards. I was in more pain than when I had started. I was throwing everything to the heavens without consideration and watching as it all came back at me and it was heart-wrenching. I was completely alone.

How do you push through a time like this? I had no clue how to muster the courage to continue to pray. Some days, things seemed so dark that even if an answer *had* come, I was likely too empty to feel it. I had no idea how to handle this strain in my heavenly communications because I had never thought it was possible; I had been taught all of my life that if I prayed and things didn't work out how I had hoped, there would be something better on the horizon. That theory may work well when you don't get into the school of your choice or you get dumped by your high school sweetheart or a slew of additional challenges but for the life of me, I couldn't make the circle of anxiety fit into that square box; if God couldn't send relief for my anxiety, what was on my horizon? Something better?

When I found myself unable to find the words my heart so desperately needed someone to hear, I got mad. Strangely, desperately mad. Not only was I trying to fight the demons of anxiety but now something that previously had been second nature to me had become all but impossible. I couldn't even fake my way through getting better by trying to pray. There was none of that. No feeling, no desire, no hope.

So, I did the next best thing I could think of – I yelled; at God, at the ceiling, at the ancestors who went before me, I don't know who exactly I was trying to get in contact with but I figured the louder I got, the greater the chance someone would finally swoop in and offer me something. I shouldn't admit it but I yelled really hateful and desperate and gnarly things about life not being fair and me not being loved and the world shrinking into a dark abyss (I wish I had the wherewithal to yell something that fantastic but it was mostly a lot of whining and complaining and sadness). I told God I had tried to live a good life and that I didn't understand (and I quote), "why he would punish me with mental illness." Yeah, I said it.

Yearly, I read one of my favorite books, "Of Mess and Moxie" by Jen Hatmaker. In it, she talks about how we each essentially have an island of untouchables – things that we hold so sacred that even God 'wouldn't dare' mess with it because it means so much. These things can be anything we hold important from kids to homes to physical health – these items are our "anything but that" exceptions that we put on our own lives. Hatmaker also points out how devastating it is when those things are messed with – the devoted mom loses a child to a terminal illness, the triathlete undergoes an amputation, the singer is diagnosed with throat cancer. But the fact remains that those things *are* messed with, they *are* tried. That, my friends, is what we call life.

Can you guess what one of the things on my untouchable island was? My mind. I've been a lot of things in my life and wore a lot of different hats but the thing I was always most sure of was my mind – its stability and resilience and logic. Come what may, I could get through it because my mind would always be stable. Read that last sentence again but this time with the irony dripping from it. My untouchable island had just been stormed as if it were Normandy. And I was a wreck.

Hatmaker goes on to talk about how it is when these islands are assaulted that we truly see what we are made of (this is obvious paraphrasing – she is much more eloquent in her description. Read the book.). It is in these moments of utmost desperation and attack on the most personal parts of our lives that we truly understand our relationship with God and what it means to surrender to Him in all things.

In the bible, we read the story of a wealthy young man who goes to Jesus and says (essentially), "I've kept the commandments, I've lived righteously, I've done all the things. What more do I have to do to have a place with you in heaven?" Jesus responds, "Go and sell all that you have and follow me." The young man had accumulated a decent amount of wealth and walked away from the Savior dejected at the weight of his task.

Many people use this story as a justification for being poor – if you have wealth or monetary riches of any sort, you can't get into heaven or, at the very least, it will be very, very difficult to do so. The young man had lived well but his wealth was preventing him from following Jesus as a disciple; translation: money makes it hard to do the right thing.

My thoughts on this parable are not in line with the above and frankly, have become much more real to me in recent months. When Jesus asks the young man to rid himself of his wealth and follow Him, He is asking him to rid himself of the one thing that stands between him and discipleship. The *one* thing. And for him, that happened to be his riches.

Each of us has a thing – like Jen Hatmaker referred to - that one sacred thing you think you'll never be asked to compromise or walk away from because (obviously) it is so important. For some of us it might be family relationships or health, for others it might be as simple as a drink or cable TV. Whatever it is that stands between us and the Savior, no matter how small or trivial it may seem, is too much. He wants us, all of us, to be His. He asks for our whole heart in order for us to have all that is His. It isn't to say we can't have things or be things or wish and dream and succeed, that isn't the message in my mind. But if those wishes or dreams don't include Him, therein lies the rub.

This proposition to give our most sacred things over to the Savior doesn't seem too difficult, especially when thought about in some future, hypothetical tense; I've given plenty of lip service to how much sacrifice I would be willing to make as long as nobody really demands it. But when you are actually brought to the front, much like the young man in the scriptures, and your island of safe treasures is called into question, it becomes so startling and frightening it takes your breath away.

I never in a thousand years would have thought I'd be asked to put my mind on the altar. Never did I think the security I'd always taken in my common sense and my ability to trust my instincts would be my sacrificial lamb. In fact, for the majority of my life, it was my logic and my reasoning that supported my entire relationship with God so having it come under attack was unbelievably unsettling.

In most Christian denominations, we base our faith off of feelings, not off of logic. We believe in Jesus Christ as the Son of God and the Savior of the World. We do this because we *feel* it, not because He manifests himself to us in the flesh. We claim miracles over happenstance because we *feel* God's hand in our lives. We love and serve and pray and fast because we *feel* something when we do.

I was never a feeler. In fact, I worried a lot about my 'feeler' being broken when I was young because everyone talked about these warm feelings that let them know there was a God, and I just didn't have them.

Don't mistake me on this though: I have always known there is a God. I know it like I know the toes on my kids' feet. But the sensation of "knowing" for me has never been that *feeling* everyone seemed so familiar with. My bosom didn't burn nor have I really ever felt that inner peace people talk about. Maybe my mind wouldn't let me, but whatever the reasoning, my "feeler" was out of fuel.

When I was in high school, my interpretation on this all changed when I heard a quote from a leader in our church who said, "Not everyone is born with a burner." Obviously, this message rang true to my heart as I still remember it to this day. My relationship with God wasn't so much about the feelings in my heart (although now that I look back, they have always been there) as it was about the clarity in my mind; I am built around logic and truth and things making sense and the concept of God has always been that for me – sensible.

This may throw some of you for a loop, especially if you are questioning the reality of a God or some higher being simply because there is no proof. But I saw 'proof' of God everywhere in my life; it made sense that life had to come from somewhere with purpose, with a past and future, that our Spirits had a connection with something greater than we could see, or why else would we love so intuitively and long for so much more than we are?

I had never been to that place of disbelief until I found myself wondering how something that was supposed to be so omniscient and merciful and good could allow me to feel so distraught. I fixated *hard* on myself and continued to pile on the self-pity and doubt until I had uprooted everything I had ever known. I was out of energy, out of faith, and out of answers.

WHERE ARE YOU, GOD?

As I continued to question the very existence of God and a Savior and mercy and prayer and all of the things I had rested on for my entire life, I decided the best thing for me was to erase all of the 'what-ifs' and 'whys' and all of the other questions that were immediately in my vision and start over.

We learn very early in our church to try to recognize the Spirit in our lives, to listen and feel and remember how it speaks to us and what that feels like. I think it is one of the strongest parts of my faith – knowing God has the capability to direct us and bless us through the guidance of His Holy Spirit. But I think, after the elementary stages of these lessons, we continue to look for that Spirit in large, marvelous ways, expecting each interaction should either be an audible voice or one that moves us to tears.

I remember sitting in my room (read: laying on my bed in the middle of the afternoon) and worrying I would never *feel* God in my life again. I knew I had felt Him before I got sick – I saw Him in big ways I could remember but for the life of me, my brain couldn't recall what it felt like on all those in-between days, the days when nothing remarkable happened but I certainly didn't feel abandoned. I prayed and plead to know who I was again, and that God was hearing me and seeing my struggle and ready to respond, and nothing happened. Not a twitch or a feeling or a curtain blowing in the breeze that was sent just for me. Just silence.

So, I tried again. Day after day, I begged God to send me a sign so that I would know He is real and aware of me and that, proverbially, He was working on things in the back of the shop. I wanted a moment, even a slight one, where I could feel overwhelmed by His grace to the point I could "recognize" it and be on my merry way with a new spring in step and God on my side. Still, nothing came.

As I sit here typing this, I can confidently say my miracle moment is still in the factory, right next to all of the miracle "prove it" moments that we read about in scripture. Luckily, mine didn't end up with me being struck dumb. And yet here I am, more confident than I have ever been that God, in fact, knows me, on a very personal and profound level and that He hears (and heard) all of those desperate prayers I threw into heaven.

So, what changed? Well, to be frank, it was me. I changed. I could go on for pages about how my relationship with my Father in Heaven has grown over the past several years with its only catalyst being confusion and fear. I could tell you about the countless people God set in my path to remind me of His love, but that at the time, I only saw as a houseguest. But what really changed is my ability to see the Spirit that I was able to recognize all those years ago, the one that moved me to tears during testimony meetings and at Especially for Youth conferences; it was sitting with me quietly, waiting for me to recognize it in a whole new way; a way that was tailored perfectly for the person I was becoming.

In the scriptures, we learn that we can distinguish the Spirit by the fruit it bears; if a plant bears up rotten fruit, the plant is deemed (for lack of a better term) bad. But if the plant bears up good fruit, it is of God. And we learn in Galatians 5:22 (KJV) that, "…the fruit of the Spirit is love, joy, peace, longsuffering, gentleness, goodness, faith…"

During the darkest times of my anxiety, I was keenly aware I wasn't feeling much of anything in my day-to-day living. I had a strong misconception God had abandoned me in my darkest hour, somehow living under the delusion that prior to me being sick, we had regular one-on-one chats about how things were going, chats where I could audibly hear His direction and understand His guidance. I can authoritatively tell you this has never been the case. I have never sat in physical council with God like you would a therapist, nor do I have a claim on faith strong enough to physically *see* Him at any point in my life.

Only now as I look back can I recognize some things I've learned about myself. First, it is easy to exaggerate my previous relationship with God when things aren't going so well – the "why have you abandoned me?" syndrome. Somewhere in the recesses of my mind, I convince myself there was a level of grandeur in my divine relationships that never actually existed, maybe because it makes my anger seem more legitimate or it gives me something (someone) to blame. The reality is my relationship with God doesn't ever change – from His side. I change. I grow closer to and farther from Him at different times in my life but like the most patient of Fathers, He sits and waits to meet me wherever I am. Fantasizing that I once knew His will for me all the time is just simply not true, and it doesn't help things. All it does is leave me questioning why He has changed rather than self-reflecting on where I've been and where I hope to get.

Second, and most importantly, God is everywhere. In our church, we frequently speak of "times" we feel the Spirit of God in our lives, like it is reserved for special occasions like girl's camp or missionary work. I think sometimes we speak of feeling the Spirit in the same sense we read about in scripture of others being *overcome* by the Spirit. This was a dangerous path for me during my anxiety because I honestly thought if I wasn't physically feeling God, He wasn't there.

I never saw visions, I never felt my heart nearly burst with love for my Savior, I wasn't moved to tears. Clearly, something was wrong.

I know now feeling God's Spirit is not reserved for special occasions. In fact, we are promised to have it literally poured out upon us as we seek for it. There is no clause in that contract, no asterisk to refer to later. It doesn't have an exception for anxiety or depression or anger or girls camp or hard days or special occasions. We have access to that blessing at all times. And when we feel love or hope or faith or empathy, charity or kindness or humility or gratitude, that IS the Spirit. That is God reminding us of who we are and what He is. And that is good.

The ironic part of not feeling God during my struggle is that He never really left, only my ability to recognize Him as His presence in my life took on a variety of new forms. I realize as I look back what I've been taught over and over again in my life: God is love. God is charity and hope and kindness and faith. And while I wasn't being moved upon by the Spirit, it was still there. It was there when I looked at my children and felt a love for them so strong that I wanted to burst. It was there when I had a kind thought about a neighbor. It was there when I got up and made dinner for my family, despite really, really not wanting to. I felt. I dare say now that I felt the Spirit the entire time I struggled through anxiety, I just didn't see it. During those months, I separated the feeling of love as not being from God, like it was just something that happened because I had *earned* it – earned the right to feel that way about my kids and my family and my neighbors.

The goodness that is God exists regardless of our earning potential, our work and sometimes even our best efforts to show Him we can stand on our own. God's willingness to bless us is not directly proportional to the number of tears we have cried over a certain topic, nor the number of nights we have laid awake or even the number of prayers we (and others) have offered in its behalf. If this were the case, mothers would never have children with broken hearts, insecurities, addiction problems or critical illness.

For too much of my life, I based my faith on results. I think a lot of us do this because that is how faith originally grows – test the seed, pray the prayers, pay the tithing, obey the commandments and *see*. The difficulty with this process comes later when we can't see. When we do the things, the tithing, the prayers, the commandments, and we still are hit by the train that we didn't see coming. This is when we start wondering, "Where are you, God?" and, "I thought if I…." and, "Why would you…" questions start permeating our prayers. These aren't bad things when they stand alone but as they become the most consuming part of our hearts, the questions take on an undertone of anger and soon, our doubts begin to absorb our faith in quick order.

I've learned over the past handful of years that we must reach a point in our lives when we realize our relationship with and faith in God can no longer be based solely on results, but only love. God doesn't withhold blessings because we haven't said enough prayers or because we missed a sacrament meeting. He doesn't allow people to get in a car accident because we forgot to specifically pray for them this morning. These things happen, the good and the bad, out of love.

God's willingness to bless us just *is* – it is an inherent part of Him that exists as sure as the sunrise. He is willing and wanting and loving us through all of it, it is just up to us to see it. Our faith, mine in particular, has to find a new foundation to be built on because the one I had, the one based on whether my life turned out how I thought it would, crumbled faster than I could have imagined when it was tested.

Trusting God does not mean everything will work out; it doesn't mean the shots will drop or the money will magically appear or that your heart will heal in the morning. Trusting God means that whether or not things work out, especially when things don't work out, He is still the one you turn to in the end. He is where gratitude flows and where sorrow is expressed. This is how foundations are built – unrelenting surrender to the process and faith that there is more to all of this than we have the capacity to understand. It feels very pie-in-the-sky, I know. But sometimes, the only place to start is with complete surrender.

There is a poignant moment in Lin-Manuel Miranda's hit Broadway musical *Hamilton* when Alexander and his wife, Eliza, have just lost their son, Philip, and are learning to, "…live with the unimaginable." In the second verse of "It's Quiet Uptown," we hear, "There are moments when you're in so deep, it feels easier to just swim down." This reflection reminds me of those endless nights with anxiety, not knowing if I had the strength to do much of anything and so, in my desperation, I found myself swimming deep into the current that kept crashing into me and taking my breath away. In the middle of my worst nights, where I found myself scared and alone and angry with God, all I could think to do was pray.

The irony is stark when I think about praying to God to help me not be angry with Him, but when desperation takes hold and your soul weeps for relief, you (I think inherently) realize there is nowhere else to turn. Even when it felt like He was silent, hope still existed that He was at least there, listening, and waiting patiently on me to surrender my whole heart to Him. I believe what that means for each of us is different. For me, it meant letting go of the idea that I could fix whatever was placed in front of me, either by my own means or even with the assistance of the divine.

Prayer doesn't always "fix" things because, simply, sometimes things aren't meant to be fixed; I firmly believe that the way things are, when we put in our best efforts and heartfelt intentions, is the way they are supposed to be, despite how ugly it may feel. Prayer is not a vehicle to fix all of the hard things that happen to us, nor is it a catch-all for all of our sorrow and pain – these things don't simply vanish as we vocalize our frustrations to whatever God we choose to worship.

So why pray? Why ask? Why plead? Why bother reaching out if not to receive some immediate blessing or, at a minimum, some sense of relief?

For me, prayer has become so much more than seeking answers or blessings, despite treating it as such for most of my life. Out of necessity, prayer became a path to accepting where I am and what I have, and seeing the beauty in where I've landed despite all my best efforts to mess that up.

Prayer is recognition that grace exists in forms both remarkable and simple.

Prayer is my verbal admission that I don't have all the answers – a fact that is both humbling and completely freeing. Prayer opens me up to others' experiences and understanding and leaves me seeking for help in all forms it may be offered.

Prayer is also an expression of hope. It is a physical tilling of the ground that exists in my heart, an exposure and a turning over of the rough parts in anticipation that something new and fresh will be planted by the Sower.

Prayer is endurance. It is rarely the quickest path to resolution, but rather the most confident one. It is the friendliest of tug-of-wars between myself and God, accompanied by a knowledge that He always aims for me to come out the victor.

Prayer is change. It is a willingness to see things how they are and admit they aren't perfect. I think it is easy for us to say this off-the-cuff and think nothing of it. But prayer is when we must truly admit our shortcomings and, if we can find the strength, ask how to change.

CHURCH

Throughout my primary battle with anxiety, going to church was rough. Really rough. The last thing I wanted to do was worship a God I felt was temporarily shunning me or see people so filled with hope while I felt like all was lost. I didn't want to hear the good news of the gospel because the only thing on my mind at that moment was survival and I most certainly didn't want to speak of the eternities when thoughts of tomorrow overwhelmed my emotions. No, going to church was not what it used to be and I legitimately questioned whether I'd ever be able to worship without a bitter taste in my mouth ever again.

But I persisted. Not because I felt like it and not because I was worried about what the neighbors would think, but simply because I didn't know what else to do. My entire life, my marriage, my job choices, my social calendar, all of it, in some way revolved around my religion and I just didn't really have a plan of what to do next. So, I did what I always do and kept things as normal as possible until I could formulate some other course of action… or until God intervened, whichever came first.

Initially, I disengaged. I was released from all of my callings (these are volunteer positions in various capacities from working with the youth to teaching Sunday school and everything in between) and took up residence in the back corner of every class I attended. I stopped participating in discussions as much, unless there was some counterpoint I felt comfortable making when someone with good intentions made a comment about God always answering our prayers. I don't know that "bitter" described my feelings at the time, but scared and sad and lonely are certainly applicable.

I think it is important to note I was certainly not alone in those feelings – getting a seat in the back row at all, let alone a corner is a true battle. It's only when you are looking for that seat that you realize how many other people are doing the same. I look back at my life and am embarrassed by how many times I mentally disregarded those people as unsocial or ornery as I made my way to the front of the class. I wonder now how many of them were using every physical muscle to stay in their seat and every mental muscle to avoid leaving the room in hysterics, just like I was during this time. Please learn from my naiveté and realize there is always someone battling their way through church and our job isn't to shame them or embarrass them through it by forcing them to comment or move in closer. Our job is simply to be glad they are there.

After several months (read: nine) of going through the motions, things started to shift ever so slightly. The interesting thing is that I can't remember a solitary moment where I was healed or where everything seemed to make sense and my faith was magically restored; it didn't happen that way. In fact, if pre-panic Carlee had a long discussion with current Carlee about their feelings on a variety of ecclesiastical topics, they would undoubtedly uncover some major discrepancies. My faith now is not the same faith I had before.

Slowly, I started feeling ok about being at church again. I felt the sarcasm and controversy slip away and make place for something new: me. Over the months of self-isolation and religious self-loathing, I figured out that my relationship with God is strictly about me and God. The end. When I was sitting in the back row of class during all of those weeks, the only thing I could focus on was what the message meant for *me* and how could it make *me* better. Not just how it would make me a better person or what I could learn from that week's sermon, but how could I use it to *heal* me? How could

God, through this hour-long discussion, heal my heart? I was so desperate for answers that I looked for this healing everywhere and became fixated on finding salve for my wounds.

Most days, especially in the beginning, I came home exhausted and no more enlightened than when I left that morning. But as I focused (and worried) and the weeks went by, I started to build some resolve about a variety of topics (both secular and spiritual) that I now hold very close to my heart. It was like I was getting clarity for the first time in my life, like I knew that the things I was feeling were specifically meant for me and regardless of the discussion or the opinions happening around me, I knew what was right for my heart.

I consider myself fortunate that through my path of reexamination and reflection, my core beliefs still reside in the basic structure of the church I've always known. Not everyone is so fortuitous – to not have to uproot their core belief system or force their changed being to fit in the framework of their current faith. Many times, scrutinizing your relationship with a higher being, particularly in the middle or just after some form of trauma, results in a total upheaval of everything previously held dear. This reexamination and reassessment don't just stop with, "What do I think is important?" but many times can cut as deep as, "Do I even believe that there *is* a God anymore?" Questions range from small perception shifts to complete paradigm overhauls. This can be a frightening undertaking for anyone who has sewn deep seeds of faith that permeate not just ritualistic beliefs and traditions but family and community life as they know it.

To those of you who don't find yourself in the same faith-filled place you once were, I see you. I'd like to say that if you just hold on long enough, everything will get back to the way it was. But it won't. It can't. Once you come to that place of self-reflection and desperation and all of those ugly things we keep ourselves from doing for so many years, you realize that going forward just as before wouldn't serve your experience the justice it deserves. Change then becomes the only way forward and in that change, hopefully, there is healing.

"Ring the bells that still can ring, forget your perfect offering. There is a crack in everything; that's how the light gets in." -Leonard Cohen

SMALL AND SIMPLE

I've noted in several parts of this manuscript that during my journey, I "noticed a small shift." This isn't unintentional, though it may seem repetitive. It is critical, if you take nothing else from my story, that you know this: there is no single answer to anxiety. Never at any point in my journey was there a miraculous moment of clarity (I'm still waiting, patiently) or resolution. I still haven't woken up at any point and only been able to hear the birds chirping. This process is long and full of tears, disfunction and confusion. It's a process I'm still going through and likely will continue through all the days of my life.

There are people who can work through anxiety, seemingly unaffected by it other than relating to other super-worriers and maybe having rules for some pretty odd stuff. I was one of those people for 36 years. Others suffer the debilitating effects of anxiety that we have touched base on in previous chapters and handfuls more that I didn't discuss, having had no experience with them myself.

What I'd like to point out here is that healing is as individual as the ailment itself. If you'll remember, I sought out information, reading a fairly clinical book about brain function and meditation and studying up on both homeopathic and medical treatments for what I was going through. Understanding gave me some peace – information and being "in the know" has always been a source of solace for me. The interesting part is that the level of information I sought out to accompany my healing could easily send someone else into a tailspin. Some of my recovery was fairly conventional;

meditation, therapy and medical intervention are all fairly common treatments for people with diagnosed anxiety and depression. Other parts of my recovery fall into the non-conventional category and certainly were nobody's recommendation except my own. I think ultimately, my body and my mind knew what we needed to heal – I just had to be able to get it to listen.

The contrast to this is in the midst of anxiety, oftentimes our rational mind shuts down and, as I've said, only focuses on survival. In that mode, our brains come up with a laundry list of things that will help us out of our funk. If you or someone you know is suffering from anxiety, it is important to know while you feel broken, your soul isn't. When seeking treatment or change or even moments of relief, trust your gut to know when things aren't right. Know that despite the tears and angst and chaos, your gut still works and has a lot to say about your healing. Trust your instincts that encourage you toward help and health. And if even that seems shaky, lean heavily on someone that can help guide you in a safe direction. In the midst of panic, this task can seem and even feel really difficult but it is critical you have someone in your corner that can give you hard no's and have hard conversations.

Sometimes while we are battling mental illness, our mind will tell us things that are counterintuitive to what you have always done and who you've always been, ways of healing ourself or bringing a temporary form of solace to a more long-term problem. Self-prescribing medication, suicide, compulsive spending, all are "outs" that can quickly take you down a road that leads away from actual recovery. Having a confident and understanding sounding board to help work through these thoughts and ideas is essential, whether it be a licensed therapist or close confidant. Be sure that you create a safe space for understanding and learning through the process, one that allows others to offer help that may be unreachable for you on your own.

CHASING PERFECTION

Sometimes, our chasing perfection leads us to forgetting who we really are and what we are capable of. Not because we aren't doing hard work, but because, ofttimes, the standards of perfection we are chasing aren't our own but rather some distant mirage, coaxing us toward a perceived happiness and peace we've only been able to dream about. It is through this relentless pursuit of someone else's dreams that we end up with a hand full of sand, right where the mirage appeared to be.

I'm not saying that goal chasing is an antiquated practice; far from, actually. I just wonder how many of our "worthwhile" pursuits are born from us, from our inner hopes and wishes for ourselves rather than dictated by the latest trend or social media phenomenon? Better yet still, how many of them came to life with the insight and approval only the Master can give, guiding us toward what we are truly meant to be and achieve?

Standards of beauty, fitness, intelligence, interest, and even baking prowess elicit emotional responses in all of us, urging us to chase someone else's ideals and leaving behind a wave of guilt when we fail to accomplish them. As I scroll (mind you, I've done this to myself), my brain is inundated with home décor I'll likely never afford and hair extensions I could never upkeep, leaving me feeling less-than as I compare myself to some else's life. It is really such a destructive cycle that study after study begs the question "why" we continue to engage in these practices.

The ironic thing is while I am out looking everywhere for fuel to add to my proverbial fire, I continue to douse it in water. Rather than searching for success and light of my own, I am surrounded and overwhelmed by the whims of others, suddenly feeling like if I don't want what they want, I can only be considered a catastrophic failure. "Why didn't we paint an accent wall?" and "Why didn't I buy those passes for my kids?" seem to plague my mind rather than a reassuring, goal-supporting narrative.

How does this chase for perfection contribute to our anxiety? Well for one, I don't recall a time when the failures of my youth had the threat of landing on a website. Trust me when I say that the 80s and 90s (that's in the 1900s, y'all, like a whole different century. I'm dead over this.) were a tough hang with our questionable fashion choices and split-level living. We did a lot of things that would make a YouTube highlight reel today but it didn't matter because after the day was done, the only evidence left behind were the memories of whoever happened to be in the room. We never got great footage of us doing dumb stuff because footage was hard to get and cameras were slow. Those were the glory days.

I worry about kids today and their fear of failure. I think the majority of it stems from a fear of being exposed – one slip up and there will be evidentiary support of their stupidity on the internet for life. Anxiety over looking ridiculous in public is what nightmares are made of now because there are literally thousands of cameras, waiting for each of us to mess up. Would I be anxious if that were the case for me when I was younger? You bet I would.

Even more than a fear of failure, I only had occasional insight into other people's successes, leading me to believe their picture-worthy days came on the same schedule as mine – a few times a year, if I were lucky (and double lucky to have the camera in focus and the pictures developed properly). Now, we take pictures to celebrate everything from waking up looking some kind of way to eating the biggest corn dog in the state. We make our entire lives out to be picture-worthy celebrations and for those folks not having a photobook kind of day or week or month, that can lead to massive amounts of social stress.

I want to make something clear before I'm tagged as the biggest hypocrite on the planet: I am a celebrating kind of gal. Big time. When I was in my early 20s, we found every reason to have a party including, but not limited to: St. Patrick's Day (I'm not Irish, nor do I drink), Christmas in July (complete with a fully-decked-out Santa Claus), and Waffice (our yearly ode to waffles and The Office, both of which should have greater air time, always). So, to rag on celebrating not only seems counterintuitive, it feels like a violation of everything I am.

I still believe in celebrating but, just like with service, you have to be doing it for the right reason. I love to see someone on social media, celebrating something they love or they have worked for. Things get a little gray though when we start posting to prove something to our followers – that we have it better than they do. Rather than celebrating for the pure joy of celebrating, we do it to fight comparisons and hold on to our share of the "good times" pie, despite the reality there is plenty to go around.

President Theodore Roosevelt once said, "comparison is the thief of joy." Teddy was light years ahead of his time, unaware that years later, we would be living in a culture of comparison, wondering why nobody was happy and feeling like our worth rested on our ability to accomplish whatever was popular or trendy at the time. My ability to fulfill other people's dreams should have no effect on my self-worth. Let's say it again, slowly. My ability to fulfill other people's dreams should have no effect on my self-worth.

I want to be very clear that the reverse is also true; other people having dreams or goals that don't coincide with my whims is also ok.

There are people who relieve stress by overhauling their physical environment. I follow a DIY-er on Instagram who talks quite often about how when she feels the anxiety monster creeping in, she grabs her paint brush and gets to work. I admire that about her because she knows what makes her tick and exactly where she can turn for solace. While her avenues are not my avenues, it doesn't make them any less valid.

In addition, it is essential as you are battling with anxiety that you stop comparing your day-to-day performance. There is a very big difference between the best you can do and the best you can do today. My best on a given day may not be the same as it was the day before, and remembering that is a path to healing. You will ebb and flow through the healing process, sometimes within hours or even minutes. Recognizing those changes and continuing to put forth your best effort each minute, regardless of what has come before, is imperative for healing and success.

EXPOSURE

Shortly after I got sick, I was asked to speak at a women's conference that was happening in our area. I said "yes" at the time, completely unaware of how shaken and unsure I would still be, nearly two months after my initial diagnosis. I had every reason to say "no" and only one reason to go ahead – I knew I had to.

To give some background, I've been a public speaker for a long time. I enjoy the connections I make through this job immensely and have never had the slightest amount of fear bearing my soul to a crowd. I especially love talking about faith and hope and confidence and gladness, so this speaking assignment was perfect for me. It gave me something to focus on as I wormed my way through my initial anxiety diagnosis and medicine trials.

Oftentimes as I sit to write out my thoughts, I am stumped as to what to say. I mull over several things for the days (sometimes weeks) leading up to a speaking engagement until the day or two before, it all kind of comes together in this magical stream of consciousness and I'm left feeling good about my direction and can proceed.

This assignment was different. I took the topic I was given and sat down to write. And I wrote. More words. More words. The thoughts continued to flow like I was the Emerson of our time. My thoughts flowed and connected and I produced enough material to not only fill my 20 minutes of allotted time but I would likely be able to remove and change a few things from session to session so I would appear interesting and charming and relaxed. I was prepared for this assignment, 100%, and had no question that I had prepared the message I was to share with these hundreds of women in my area.

You always know that when a story starts like this, the conflict or the main character's fall from grace is pending, right? And oh, how she fell.

The day of the conference I woke, well, in the hot mess I had been in for the previous 45 days or so. I didn't sleep much the night prior. I was nervous – sick nervous, and couldn't stop crying as I got ready. I had invited my mom to come to the conference to hear me speak and bless her for not sliding over three seats when we got there because I was in a state. My palms were sweaty and I cried one tear at a time as we sat in the back during a keynote speaker. Her message was tender, of course. But nothing that should have induced that level of watershed or panic. I was full blown nervous about something that should have been my "thing".

As the clock ticked on and doom inched closer, I pulled myself together and made one final pass through my notes. None of them made sense. I couldn't seem to connect one idea to the next and everything felt really blurry – mentally. My eyes were blurry, yes, but you know those times when you are sure that you've got a hold of something and the world turns sideways and nothing looks the same? No? Just me? Well, it happened.

As I stood in front of the first breakout session of the conference, I slowly started into my notes, dropping generalities and a few thoughts I knew that stood on solid ground. And that took about six minutes. And at that moment, once all of the notes had basically been devoured and all of the words I had written and had poured out of me were gone, I was left alone. And I knew exactly what I had to do.

During this time, my two babies were very young, seven and four, to be exact. We did a lot during those years but like a lot of moms, I spent a good portion of my free time watching (read: listening while I did something else) kids' movies. One of our favorites during this period was Disney's Moana. There is a part in the story where Moana is on her boat and she looks at the sea and asks for help on her journey to find Maui, the great warrior, and restore the heart of Tafiti. As she speaks to the sea, a great storm arises and sends Moana and her boat into chaos; the boat is overturned and she wakes up, sandy and alone, with a broken boat, on a beach somewhere. Moana angrily addresses the sea with, "Um… what?! I asked you to help me and you destroyed my boat!" Moana is not a happy island dweller.

Moana had been through a lot, literal rough seas. She was angry after asking for help and essentially getting her entire plan destroyed. But what Moana didn't know at the time is that the sea had dropped her right where she needed to be – right on the same island as the infamous Maui. But all she could see in that minute was the hard.

I relayed this story to the women at this conference and then began to speak to them about how I was in the middle of my own storm, one that without question would change my direction, my life, forever. And right now, I was mad. I was frustrated that despite thinking I was on my own noble journey, and despite asking for help, a storm had been set off and was raging all around me. I was gasping for air and being pulled downward.

I spoke of my anxiety battle and the fact that I, while not being very far into it, was already terrified of what was to come. I spoke of therapy and medicine and prayer and anger and sadness. In case you were curious, this was *not* the topic I was assigned.

But at the tail end of my talk, I was able to hold on to something so precious that it still sits with me today. And if I were the only one to grasp onto this lesson during my time at the conference, then I guess that was the point. But the lesson is this: there is always hope. Despite not being able to come up for air and despite the clouds looking dark for as far as I could see, I had hope that in the end, just like Moana, the storm would drop me right where I needed to be.

Whether it was garnering empathy for those with similar struggles, learning how to be less judgmental, or simply understanding why it is important to take care of myself, my storm and your storms have a purpose. Always. And while it may feel like you are drowning, you will be given enough opportunities to surface, take a breath, and fight on until you come to the place you are supposed to be.

2020

It was *early* March of 2020 and my mom and I had arrived in Vegas for our annual trip to the PAC-12 Women's Basketball Tournament. This was our third year attending the tournament and it always is one of my favorite weekends of the year.

During our second night at the hotel, I woke up to my heart racing and my head pounding so hard that I was unsure of where I was. I hadn't been dreaming so having a sudden onset of the symptoms seemed odd. I got up and walked to the bathroom, hoping a shift in position or posture would alleviate things and I would be able to calm down. But it didn't work. As I laid back down, my heart continued to race and I started to become nauseous. I became more and more restless as I was unable to sleep, wondering what had caused my body to go into such a ruckus.

At this point in time, I had been off of my anxiety medication for roughly eight months and while I occasionally had bouts with very mild depression or nerves, I hadn't encountered anything my weighted blanket couldn't fix. But this felt different, and frighteningly familiar. And I wasn't prepared for what was to come.

The minute we landed back home, the world shut down. There was a mysterious virus that had made its way to the United States and started spreading in and around Washington state. While we were on our trip, Utah identified its first case of Covid-19 and was beginning to close; large office buildings in Salt Lake City were desolate and the freeways abandoned as the entire world grappled with sickness and death and unknown transmission of a mysterious illness. It felt really heavy.

On the morning of March 18, 2020, after a couple of weeks of bleaching everything in sight and trying to understand what was coming our way, my husband was up and getting ready to leave the house for the day and I was already feeling antsy about whether or not he had enough hand sanitizer. The kids were asleep and I had just gotten up to use the restroom and was on my way to get dressed when we heard a very loud gush of wind pass by the window. When the wind didn't stop and the floors began to sway back and forth, we knew we were in the center of something very different than an abnormally strong windstorm. Trevor rushed to grab the kids while I stood in shock, trying to convince myself that if this was the end, at least we were all together. (To be fair, I haven't been through many earthquakes before. Oh, and that fear of dying thing I've discussed at length, well, apparently, I wasn't as "cured" as I thought.)

At 7:09 that morning, Northern Utah experienced a 5.7 magnitude earthquake that left everyone in a frenzy. Once the house stopped swaying, we grabbed our laptops and chargers, our emergency paperwork, and our 72-hour kits and loaded them into the car. We backed the car out of the garage, thanks to a quick-thinking neighbor who reminded us that garage doors may not open if we suffer a sizable aftershock and power went out or the door was damaged in any way. (Do yourself a favor and find a neighbor like this. It will help *almost* as much as a therapist.) And then we sat and waited for things to get worse.

Emergencies are never pleasant but for someone with anxiety, they can be horribly triggering, mostly due to the hysteria that surrounds them. People with OCD and anxiety generally cling to control and calm and the events following a catastrophic event aren't exactly that. I'll admit this was not my best day as I read news report after news report and just cried. My husband received an ill-timed text from a well-intentioned contact that "they" (the powers that be in natural disasters) were expecting a 9.0 aftershock within the hour and that, my friends, was enough to start running worst-case scenarios through my mind as we sat in our kitchen and waited on Mother Nature to show us her vengeful side. (Just for your reference, and for mine the next time an earthquake strikes, this is NEVER true. Such things can't be predicted and it would take a very, very incredible act of God (totally capable) for a 9.0 earthquake to happen on Utah's fault line; just not big enough. Exhale.)

Without trying to sound dramatic (it just comes naturally, I guess), this was one of the most emotional and mentally taxing days of my life. I sat at my kitchen table, post-earthquake, with my laptop open, toggling back and forth between the Utah news coverage of the earthquake and Governor Andrew Cuomo's daily news brief about what the state of New York was doing to prepare for the influx of infections and deaths from the Corona Virus. The previous week, we had been notified that our kids would be out of school for at least two weeks, most likely unable to return for the remainder of the year and we would need to home school them full-time. Our car was packed, our emergency resources ready and waiting. The freeways were closed because of the earthquake, people were dying of a mystery illness, and I was lost; to be confused and scared and under-resourced and worried about my kids, our parents, our siblings and their families just felt like too much. I was worried about the ground opening and the toilet paper supply all over the course of eight seconds.

This time though, the worries weren't made up. Very real, very scary things were happening that made a lot of otherwise calm people feel very anxious. But thankfully (now, sort of), the feelings were very familiar. I had seen this and felt it before and knew that if I didn't take an immediate step back, I was going to be in a world of hurt. After several days of introspection and trying to convince myself I didn't need any more help, I made an appointment with Dr. S and that's when he spoke about healing injuries and we made a longer-term plan for my anxiety medication. As I sit here now, over two years after the trauma (read: 2020) began, I feel nothing but gratitude for both an understanding doctor and therapist who taught me how to recognize the alarm bells before they grew too loud.

2020 was a beast of epic proportions for everybody. In fact, I think it was the straw that broke the proverbial backs of a lot of people suffering with mild mental illness. Loneliness, worry, uncertainty, financial instability… the list goes on of the catastrophic mental weight we all bore during the worldwide pandemic. "Trauma" became a regular part of all of our vocabulary as we looked to navigate our way back to a new normal and anxiety became a much more common part of our daily living than it had ever been. Perhaps that is what made me feel safe enough to write this memoir, I don't know.

Regardless of what you've faced over the last two years, anxiety has made a comeback of epic proportions in the public eye; people whose brand is happy-go-lucky have brought their mental health struggles into the light, exposing what many of us have fought with for years but were afraid to recognize. And while I'm certainly not grateful for the pain and suffering and confusion brought on by a worldwide pandemic, I can be grateful for that.

2020 was a lot of things for my mind and my life, a statement I'm sure we could all embroider on a pillow and have it make perfect sense to each person who reads it. One critical thing that came into perspective for me over that time and in the subsequent time since then is the value in knowing my limits. It is ok to recognize when you need a timeout. It is ok to guard your mental health like a fortress and to shut the gates when it is time for a break. It is ok to admit (even out loud if you need to) you aren't handling things and may need some help.

In October 2002, Elder Joseph B. Wirthlin of the Quorum of the Twelve Apostles of The Church of Jesus Christ of Latter-Day Saints delivered a powerful address to a churchwide general conference titled, "Shall He Find Faith on the Earth" that I think of often. He tells a story of years ago when he noticed the light all around him seemed to be fading; despite replacing bulbs and lamps, he was finding it difficult to read in the dim light they provided. He finally made an appointment with an ophthalmologist who examined his eyes and diagnosed him with a cataract in his eye. He makes a poignant statement near the end of his story by saying, "The light had never diminished; only my capacity to see the light had been lessened." Once he was able to put his eyes in capable hands, the cataract was corrected and light, again, flooded his sight.

I love this story and reference it in a variety of circumstances in my life. It is particularly significant to me as I discuss my battle with anxiety and panic because of the way I felt about seeking help and medical intervention for my issues. I had heard story after story of people being put on anti-depressants and it "messing up" their personality or their ability to function. Despite being a mental mess in the moment, I didn't want to lose who I was because of a pill.

I realize now that with proper dosing and monitoring, my medication actually helped me to become the *real* me I hadn't seen in ages, not a version of me, shrouded in worry and fear. The medication I was on helped to curb the intrusive thinking that had progressively gotten worse (nearly unmanageable) over the years and to see things as they really were. I wasn't lost. I had just temporarily lost the ability to see myself for who I really was. And the combination of medication and therapy eventually brought my sight back into focus.

Making a medical parallel with this story is the easy part and one that seems to make the most sense. But the parallel that is more important for me, the one that is harder to tell, is about self-recognition and seeking help.

Generally speaking, the majority of people who struggle with the ailments I have are very organized, efficient, high-functioning, responsible, type-A personalities. I speak from experience when I say this: we don't like to ask for help. We are efficient self-starters, list-makers and "to-do"-ers who struggle to delegate and thrive in responsibility. It is easy, even habitual, to continue to take on more than we can handle. I'll admit I ignored the signs of burn-out for years, probably because it was never on my list of things to plan for so clearly, if it wasn't on the list, it wasn't happening. (I'm fully aware of how ridiculous this is, but it's true).

You can imagine my dismay when I found myself out of control and unable to do *anything*, let alone the things that had made the list. I certainly didn't want to admit I was drowning or even struggling for air. It took me too long to recognize things weren't as they should be, longer than was safe for me and my family. That is a regret I'll live with for the rest of my life.

I'm going to make a statement I wouldn't have been willing to make three years ago: there is no shame in waving the white flag when you feel like things aren't right. And just because it looks like everyone around you is living "full steam ahead" doesn't mean that is true. It takes some time and self-awareness to examine how you are feeling. There is no emotional barometer to tell you if things are "off"; our "not right" is solely based on your own scale, not on anyone else's ability to function.

In The Book of Mormon, we read an admonition from the Prophet Alma to the people as he speaks of repentance. He says, "And now behold, I say unto you, my brethren, if ye have experienced a change of heart, and if ye have felt to sing the song of redeeming love, I would ask, can ye feel so now?" (Alma 5:26).

I often use this as a gauge on how I'm doing – not just in my repentance but in my basic pursuit of joy. I know what it feels like to be happy and to feel at peace, I've felt it before and know what that looks like for me. So, I simply ask myself, "…can I feel so now?" If the answer is a resounding, "no way," I know it is time to make some space for my mental health and examine what is keeping me from that stillness. Sometimes, it is simply a rough day and a fresh start does the trick. Other times, finding that peace requires the elimination of things, or even people, out of my daily living. Regardless of the steps I take, Elder Wirthlin's prompt continues to ring true, time and time again – the light has never faded, only my ability to see it.

RECOVERY

What does it mean to recover? Well, according to the trusted dictionaries I could reference, it means to return to a state of health, mind or strength; recuperation; healing; rallying; a comeback; the *process* of getting better. I like that last phrase – a process. Because to tell you that I have "recovered" from anxiety would be less accurate than to say I am *recovering* from anxiety, and fully tuned-in to the fact that the process might look like more of an eternal one than I had hoped.

I, like many of us, have become more and more expectant of instant gratification and resolution in my life, so much so that when large, looming problems or worries work their way into my view, I find myself looking for the nearest exit. I don't know that I am scared of them necessarily, but I am quick to force a resolution that will "resolve" things as quickly and quietly as possible. My anxiety diagnosis was no different. I had absolute plans to have this little inconvenience packed up in a box and shipped off in quick order.

I listened to a wonderful podcast recently, discussing how God works in our lives and the struggle many of us have in adjusting to His timetable. The featured guest on the show said something that struck me to the core; he said we shouldn't make the assumption that God works in an instant, rather than through a process. I recognize that I've spent much of my trial wondering when my "miracle moment" will come and I will emerge from the lion's den like Daniel of old, victorious over my trial and my fears left safely behind me. How much healthier and healing it could have been to give God time rather than expecting instant restoration; time to plan, time to orchestrate, even time to mourn with me, as we are so often instructed to do.

I believe God does that, mourns with us. I believe sometimes He leaves us sitting in the dark for a minute *so that* He can sit beside us and weep. I believe He does this with a gentle palm in the center of our backs, not forcing us ahead but allowing us a reassuring reminder He is right there.

I believe before my anxiety, I almost got so used to God's omnipresence that I forgot the touch of His hand in my life, that I failed to see Him guiding me along my very personal path, but it's there. It is one thing to know God is almighty and all-knowing, it is a very different thing to see it. I spent so much time resting on my comfortable laurels, knowing whatever happened in my life must be "the plan" or "everything happened for a reason" that I never stopped to recognize *why* it was my plan, *what* was my reason.

Another definition of "recover" I have drawn close to outlines a process of regaining possession or control of something lost or stolen. There are times when I feel like this definition is more suitable for those suffering from depression and anxiety; the idea that something profoundly sacred has been taken from them rings true, over and over again, as they seek to find a happiness and a peace that once existed – one they likely took for granted until it was no more. For me, it's the word "lost" that seems to mark my journey best.

I remember attending my husband's office party nearly a year after my initial diagnosis. I had been several months off of my anxiety medication at the time and this was a first major outing (read: not grocery store run) for me since that transition. We were at a lovely dinner party with his co-workers at a swanky hotel in downtown Salt Lake. I remember the ride to the party and how with every passing block, my anxiety seemed to creep higher and higher until, at the parking garage, it seemed to have a full grip on my neck.

We made our way upstairs and the last thing I really remember about the rest of that night was throwing up in the bathroom and spending the remainder of the evening living in my own personal cone of silence.

This sounds like a spring-break-gone-bad story but I can assure you that I did not imbibe at any point in the evening. As I've discussed, anxiety can come with a wide range of side effects and one of mine was stomach pyrotechnics; I spent a good portion of my time studying toilet bowls all around town so if you ever need a restroom recommendation, I'm your huckleberry.

That entire night, we were surrounded by perfectly lovely people in a safe environment and I just couldn't get out of my head. If memory serves, there was music and food and, most likely, fantastic conversation, and I sat with a death grip on Trevor's leg during all of it. (He has feeling back, so don't go feeling sorry for him.) There was no trigger, no run-in with the police, not even bad hors d'oeuvres I could blame the panic on, it just came like a tidal wave crashing onto shore. I spent the evening in a fog, pining for my sweatpants and blankets while discussion continued about holiday plans and family outings.

As I remember the brevity of that evening, I still feel really angry, like I was robbed of something really important. Not that I find work parties particularly important, but as I reflect on that evening, what I regret is the *time* I can't ever get back. This was the second holiday season after my initial breakdown and I was still trying to figure out how to cope. I couldn't get excited for my kids and all of their holiday hopes, I couldn't support my husband at his work function, I couldn't even get out of a parking garage without convincing myself everything would be ok.

Anxiety is a thief who shows no remorse; it takes time and attention away from things that really matter and drowns them in a sea of self-pity and sorrow. It fills the air with angst and silence and robs it of joy and laughter. This holiday party and so many other occasions fall into the void of that time where I was sick and my heart hurts for every second.

Anxiety also takes seemingly ordinary things and makes them very difficult. Enjoying the yearly holiday celebrations is one of a laundry list of things that are still incredibly difficult for me to do as I recover from my anxiety. Other seemingly ordinary things are still triggers for me that hash up uncomfortable memories of anxious days; these include sitting in my living room for extended periods of time, driving past the hospital where I received treatment, passing a hotel where Trevor and I stayed when I was sick, and unfortunately, taking a hot bath. All of these everyday activities put my mind into a bit of a tailspin when I encounter them, one that takes more than a few minutes to reconcile.

But then I remember this is a journey and recovery is about taking back possession of something that was lost or stolen. In those minutes of uncertainty, I can choose to either let anxiety continue to steal precious moments from my mind, or I choose control. Exposure therapy has played a major role in my ability to face all of the things I still fear and create a new reality for myself. I can either continue to let anxiety take moments or I can really harness recovery and re-take command of my own time. It is a decision I don't always come out on the right side of, but it is happening more frequently and more quickly each time I work through it.

When I was young, my mom taught me sewing lessons. I am by no means an expert but I loved to watch her sew and learning the basics from her is something I will always remember. And while I love to create new things, I find sewing has its most utility in mending, fixing the old. You see when something is mended, it goes from a broken or torn state to being usable again. As I've seen it, the item is generally put back together even stronger than it originally started. Why? Well because its weakness has been exposed and the hope is the Mender can reinforce that weak spot to avoid a future tear. He or she takes into account the material, the stress, the environment and fixes the item in a way that will not only repair the hole or tear but in a way that will prevent it from happening again. That's not to say that other tears can't occur but for now, that spot is safe, whole, usable.

The other thing I find interesting about mending is if you look hard enough, you can usually see it. A jacket that has been mended usually has a tightly-woven line of thread that runs through its previous tear, almost like a scar. While it is visible, you can almost tell this line is a mark of strength in the garment, a place where it has been reinforced. I think these marks give an item character, a story to be told for years to come about all that it has been through.

Broken, torn things need mending, me included. While the process is difficult, it can be really transformative. These sacred places that have been torn open in my soul the last two years have been painful and visible and unsightly. But as I focus on healing and understanding and change, I can feel those tears coming back together again, stitch by stitch. These gaps I've stared at for so long, the weak points in my life are becoming stronger, reinforced I suppose, until hopefully, they become whole again. The changes are visible, maybe even apparent to some. But they no longer bother me. They are my character, my story.

Today, more than ever, I am grateful for the Master Tailor who sees the value in my offering, as imperfect as it will continue to be. It would have been easy to discard the scraps I've brought to His table as garbage, unworthy of salvation. But that's why He is the Master – He sees what others can't and recognizes the value of each piece. Only He can take into account the stress and the material and the environment and make His repairs, all the while making me into something more suitable and sturdier than I was to begin with.

To Him, my offering is enough. Never perfect, but always enough.

THE DANCE

Anxiety and depression are a quiet battle, taking place in the sacred spot that connects your heart and your head. To this day, in fact, I don't know that anyone outside of my immediate family knows the entirety of the struggle I faced; hospital visits and medication aren't exactly an uplifting dinner topic when you are out with friends. While my family was a tremendous support during my initial confrontation with anxiety and panic (they still are), the loneliness I felt still plagues my memory more than anything else.

In my front room, I had two oversized chairs that flanked our window that became a primary spot for my worrying. They looked to the southwest where, past the houses on our street, there is a large nature reserve and mountains in the distance. The open land contains high, dry grasses and shrubs and are often teaming with the sounds of the small birds who make their home there. While my husband was at work, I'd sit in one of those chairs, trying to vanquish thoughts of death, and just watch the sky. Sometimes it only lasted minutes as the tug of littles and their needs often interrupted the silence. Other times, as the kids played in the yard, I could sit for an hour and just stare past the houses to the fields. Generally, they were quiet and the minutes passed without interruption or movement. But every now and again something, a strong breeze or maybe a lurking animal I couldn't see, would rustle up the grasses and send those birds into flight. It was as if, all at once, chaos erupted and hundreds of birds filled the sky in a swarm of tumult and terror. They would lift and dodge and swarm and move until they knew it was safe to rest again. For minutes, the sky turned dark with uncertainty and commotion and just as quickly as it seemed to begin, all was quiet.

Watching the birds in flight was always fascinating for me and never seemed to get old. Once the birds rose from the grass, they moved in unison, creating a wave of darkness that almost seemed orchestrated, like someone was pushing and pulling strings attached to each one. As they flew, they created graceful patterns in the sky, even in the midst of unsettling moments in their day. Eventually, the birds came to rest again and peace was restored.

As I think back about these birds, it seems easy to draw a parallel to my own life, one that I missed while they were merely a distraction. Sometimes, just when things seem peaceful and calm, something unexpected causes sheer turmoil in our lives. Like the birds escaping inclement weather or a vivacious animal, we take off in a rush to find safety. Everything looks and feels chaotic and urgent as we try and locate a safe place to land. I'm sure for the birds, nothing feels good about being in the center of a dark swarm.

But from a distance (in my case, hindsight), we can see a pattern forming, a dance, that looks like something or Someone else is in absolute control, urging us up and down, side to side, and teaching us to follow the lead. From a distance we see the patterns forming, thick and thin, and the miraculous way the flock moves in unison to some rhythm that only their souls can recognize; something beats deep within them and begins to make sense of the chaos. There is no longer fear or trepidation, just a return to what they were born to do. They escape the impending threat and simply fly.

On the opposite wall from those oversized chairs hung my favorite picture of the Savior. He has an almost imperceptible smile and unquestionable sense of peace in His face. When it was dark and I could no longer see the fields, I would often turn and look at that picture, silently praying for light or some sense of relief from myself.

I spent so much time staring into His face that it is (I hope) permanently etched into my mind.

Only now that I think back about the hours that I spent staring out that window do I realize something so profound: I wasn't alone watching those birds. God was there, giving me moments of exhilaration and peace, reassuring me I would feel again. He provided this incredible focal point for me to hold on to through the really troubling days of uncertainty and fear. Watching those birds rise and fall in grace and beauty gave me hope I might be able to do the same, one day.

But also, the Savior, sitting quietly over my shoulder, patiently waiting with me through my distractions until it became too dark to see. It was then I had to turn and face Him, always steady and always waiting, and plead for guidance and direction. He was there through all of it, but I always noticed Him more in the dark. When it was just us, me and Him, no distractions, no other place to turn, I found myself intently focused on Him. I wondered if He knew me. I wondered if He saw past my un-showered exterior and heard my heart crying out for peace. His immovable presence on my wall became almost lifelike as I spoke my deepest fears out loud to only Him, yearning for understanding and longing for grace.

In the scriptures (Matthew 10, KJV) we read that a sparrow is sold for a farthing (very, very cheap) and yet not one of them falls from the sky without the Father being intimately aware. He knows us and will compose the most beautiful sonnets, even in (especially in) our trials *if* we trust Him enough to take the lead. The center of the storm will inevitably seem dark but I can assure you that you are a beautiful part of the dance.

"Fear ye not therefore," the scripture tells us, "ye are of more value than many sparrows." (Matthew 10:31, KJV).

FINAL THOUGHTS

My story may or may not sound familiar to you; thousands and thousands of people have run-ins with crippling anxiety each day. It is a journey that is utterly personal and completely terrifying. It is a battle I wouldn't wish on my worst enemy, and, oddly enough, one I wouldn't walk back.

Throughout my writing process these past couple of years, I've written down some things that have felt important but had a tough time working their way into the manuscript. So, this is the chapter every author feels like they have to add at the end, either because they forgot something (me) or are afraid some things in their story might not have made much sense (also me). Regardless of the reason, here we are. At the risk of sounding needy, I hope you will indulge me in a few final thoughts:

To Them

For those of you who are living with someone who suffers from anxiety and/or mental illness, I say 'thank you'. Thank you for your patience and love and support as we try to navigate the darkest recesses of our minds. I want you to know that many times, our biggest fear is making life harder on you and there is an extreme sadness that accompanies the thought of disappointing or frustrating the people we love the very most. None of this makes sense to us either, so navigating it with an extra hand on our shoulder means the world.

While deep down we know that your most perfect intention is to get us back to what we once were, be mindful of how you encourage.

This is not a problem you can "fix". Telling an anxiety sufferer to just think happy thoughts is not a prescription for healing. Telling someone not to be sad because it could be worse is like telling them not to be happy because things could be better. It just makes no sense. Letting people sit in their feelings and actually *feel* them is a critical step to processing anxiety and depression. Please don't try to force anyone into happiness. Cookies won't do it (they help though, hand to the square, they help) and neither will a book on self-esteem. Eventually, they may offer much-needed guidance but don't expect it to solve any issues overnight. In my experience, it took multiple channels of help and, most importantly, time, to even begin healing.

That being said, be mindful of how long your loved ones are struggling. I was once told that feelings are like seasons: all of them are good and have their place but it's when you stay in one too long that there is a problem. If weeks and months pass without reprieve, it may be time to check in and make sure they are doing ok and are aware of the resources available to help them fight this war.

This is a process, a tough one, but one that *will* get better. Do your best to remind your loved one to take care of themselves. Give them space and time to meditate or to talk or to cry. Give yourself space and time to meditate or to talk or to cry. In the thick of this battle, everyone needs to communicate openly and honestly about their feelings of overwhelm and grief. Secretly harboring feelings of bitterness or frustration will not help. Communicate. That is enough.

Hug if you must.

When I was really sick, I could tell my dad was really struggling to make heads or tails of what was happening with me and why I was not just *happy*. He didn't push, but I could tell that he didn't understand all of the moving parts in my life and just wanted to fix things for his kid. As time went on, he and my mom would watch and read things about anxiety and people who suffered from it (there is no shortage of material on this, particularly from 2020) and they would occasionally speak with me about what they saw or they would save interviews on their DVR for me to watch; I found the information helpful and, in a non-intrusive way, felt like they were interested in truly understanding what was happening.

One day, my dad showed up at my house and said he had watched a segment about giving eight-second hugs and how it helps to suppress your nervous system and helps to reduce your blood pressure, even temporarily. In the middle of my driveway, my dad hugged me with a conviction I will never forget – like if he just held onto me long enough, all of this would just melt away. And I just exhaled. Eight seconds is a long time on a bull, but longer in a desperately-needed gesture. I won't ever forget the care and concern my dad conveyed for me that day; I still lean on it when things are hard. Just knowing someone would literally hug it out in order to make sure you are ok is a gift. Remember that.

This last bit of information is going to feel heavy, despite my intentions for the opposite. Restoration, in its truest form, may not be possible for the person that is struggling. They may not ever be exactly as you see them in your mind's eye nor may they ever return to their former glory. And while that may feel disappointing, I can promise you it is good. Returning to how things were is a restoration of the unhealthy and broken. Breathe deep in this process and encourage growth and change. The goal is to come away from this changed for the better. Lean into it and allow for discovery, not just for the person that you love but for yourself.

The Kids

This is a topic I can't write about without severe emotional heartache so I plan to keep this very brief: I had two kids who sat with me through my battle with anxiety, both of them very young. I still dream about the amount of therapy I might have caused them during this time of their lives... and then I watch them run off with their friends and realize everything is going to be ok.

Kids are RESILIENT little buggers who are generally more in-tune with emotions than we can be as adults. My kids spent a lot of time in bed with me, snuggling and watching movies while I slept or read or tried to get my life in order. Are they worse for it? No. In fact, those times with my kids tucked in by my sides are some of my most prized and sacred memories.

I talk fairly openly with my kids about my anxiety and let them know when I am having a hard time. They are aware that different problems affect different people in a variety of ways. They have been able to see I'm human and can crumble with the best of them. They are empathetic and caring and good and some of the best salve for the soul.

Am I writing this to take away some of my own guilt? Maybe. But I still find it true – bring your kids on your journey with you. You don't have to show them all of the late nights and crying, but letting them see you are fallible is so critical to you both surviving this intact. Kids need to see that you can do hard things – I promise you this will not be their only run-in with anxiety so coach them while you can.

To You

For those of you suffering with mental illness, whether it be anxiety or depression or any of the myriad of issues we face: healing is work. Constant work. It is unbelievably easy to slip back into old habits and to forget to take care of yourself. Staying healthy is a constant job; between exposure work, meditation and other forms of self-care, it can almost be exhausting. Don't stop. Reassess frequently. If it is easy, you aren't doing it right.

I'm two years back on my daily anxiety medication and finally able to discuss it openly with others. No, I still don't want to be the pill-popping heroine of anyone's tale; I haven't come *that* far or become *that* delusional. But I'm not ashamed of my diagnosis nor am I ashamed of my journey. Every morning that I rendezvous with my medication, I take just a quick second to breathe out the bad and pull in the good; for me it has become more than swallowing a pill that unquestionably makes up for shortcomings in my wiring. Now, that holy moment every morning is a reminder of where I was and how far I've been able to come. Taking anxiety medication isn't glamorous, but neither is not getting out of bed for weeks at a time because of crippling sorrow.

Remember that every day, sometimes every hour, is the start of a new path. Please don't compare yourself to the "pre-anxiety" you – it never works out because despite thinking that you were "better" then, you really weren't. Focus on this minute, then this hour, then this day. Today's best may not be what it was yesterday and that is perfectly fine. It is never about the speed, but rather all about the direction. And as long as you are facing healing and hope, you will make it.

One week during my recovery phase, I attended the Latter-Day Saint Ogden Temple with my husband. Before I got sick, the temple was a place I could go to reflect on life and find some peace in the midst of chaotic parenting and work. After I got sick, the temple was a crowded place full of process and time expectations and struggle for me. But to try and find my old self, we made a "go" of it and went to spend some time there.

As I was sitting and waiting, I quickly became overwhelmed by my surroundings. I had been having my own private wrestles with God and now sitting here in His house felt daunting. There were people and my dress felt tight and it was so hot and why did everyone around me know I was freaking out?! Ok, they didn't. But it felt like it.

I finally couldn't take it anymore and got up to slide out the side of the chapel, the place where we wait before going on to do more of our temple work. As I stood, I saw a temple worker reach her hand out and pull me off to the side, just gently and quietly, while other temple patrons passed. As we stood there, holding hands, she let others make their way past me until the room was empty. At that point, this lovely woman turned to me and said, "You know, I grew up on a farm. And my dad had a lot of equipment. And he taught me to drive that equipment. And you know what he always reminded me? Every vehicle has brakes for a reason." She smiled and hugged me and led me out to a more private area where Trevor and I could just sit.

Every vehicle has brakes for a reason. We are given the ability to stop and readjust when we need to. Pumping the breaks isn't bad, it is part of who we are! Brakes provide a safety and a security we all need, allowing us to reassess our surroundings and then move forward when it is safe. That reassessment time is critical to moving forward with any sort of mental illness, despite feeling like full-throttle might get us to our objective quicker. Pump the brakes and see what clarity that can bring. Slow and steady, slow and steady. You can do this.

AFTERWORD

It has been just over three years since I was originally diagnosed with generalized anxiety disorder and intrusive thinking and in general terms, my life is very much the same as it was before; I'm still married (although when I think back about all of the ugly crying and turmoil I heaped on my husband, I sometimes wonder how!), my kids are getting older and we are doing the normal "family" things like swimming lessons and vacations and homework. I attend church and visit my parents and catch a drink with my friends when time allows.

On the flip side, my life, the interior one I live with every day, is notably different than what it was before my diagnosis; I'm more skeptical, I don't laugh as often, and my sleep is still a work in progress. On hard days I can cry easily for no apparent reason and I have to be hyper-aware of my mental health, recognizing when I'm overloaded and need to take a breather. It has become one of the few things in my life that requires a watchful eye and constant protection. All of these things are the "not-my-favorite" side-effects of the battle I've been through, but ones I think will get better with time – I'm working on them every day.

I don't write this to drip additional despair on this narrative, nor to publicize my personality flaws that seem to have risen to the surface over these past couple of years. Nor do I write this to let you know how self-aware I've become and try to convince you that I know all of the answers. Far from it.

I wanted to write about the fact that things still aren't "great" because that is the reality. For sure I am having many more good days than bad, a truth that never escapes my attention. I am grateful as I work and strive to be better, that God's grace has swooped in and allowed me to feel again. I see so much of what I once was in my day-to-day actions and abilities that I can't help but hope for brighter days ahead.

At the same time, I have a very personal relationship with the fact that this might be as good as it gets. My hope beyond hope is that I'm not going through all of this just to come out the other side the exact same person who went in. Unfortunately, some of the characteristics I picked up along the journey are not all roses and I am learning to deal with my new found Doubting Thomas who has settled into the recesses of my mind.

I do, however, cling to the hope that even if this is as good as it gets *for now*, that is still quite remarkable. The fact is, I did a really hard thing. And I continue to slay that dragon with each step I take forward.

In the beginning, I mentioned a cultural hyper-focus on the eternities and perfection that make it really difficult to live in the "now". That chase has been a contributing factor to all I've mentioned in this memoir. But it is that same hyper-focus on the forever that only now brings hope; one day, all will be made right. I know this to be true. Whether it is anxiety and depression, OCD and intrusive thinking, psychosis or a myriad of other physical, mental or social issues, I know that this isn't forever. There is so much more to this life than this, there is so much more to me than this. And every day I stretch for forever and whatever that might hold, is one day closer to eventual rest.

We speak of heaven and all that it has to offer there and I wonder sometimes what that physically looks like. But the more I've worked to understand my purpose through all of this, the more I recognize that heaven, for me, is a feeling. I feel it when I look at my kids and remember their resilience through all of this. Man, they are awesome. I feel it when gratitude floods my heart that I am still here; it is especially strong in the early hours of the morning as I greet a new day and add another "made it" check mark to my calendar. I feel it in the small acts of service from those who are fighting their own battles and my wonder at how they do it. And for a moment, I know what it feels like to be whole again. And my best day will be when that feeling comes to stay. That will be heaven.

ACKNOWLEDGEMENTS

I want to thank each of you for reading and sharing this memoir. Writing something so personal has been a dauting task made much easier by the encouragement sent to me along the way. I'm forever grateful to those of you that have been willing to share your stories as I have worked to share mine. As I've had the opportunity to speak about my journey, countless numbers of you have been brave enough to say, "Me, too" or "My daughter..." or "I have a friend", all of which have given me the courage to continue forward in vulnerability and truth. Thank you for your strength and your honesty.

To my parents who fought so hard to understand what was going on with me, and who loved me hard even when they didn't understand: thank you. Thank you for giving me a bed to sleep in, phone calls every day, and long, awkward hugs. Thank you for encouraging healing by simply being there. Thank you most for loving my babies when I felt like my offering wasn't enough.

To my editing crew: Trevor, Debbie, Jan, Steve and Lisette, you are all rocks in my life. Your support and feedback are what every person deserves in their sphere. Heaven only knows how glad I am to have it in mine.

There are countless people that I hope to thank one day that, knowingly or not, helped me breathe another day and silently, over the course of several years, cheered me on through their perfectly-timed miracle moments in my journey. From sharing scriptures to dropping off vuuuury large sodas to writing a note on a napkin after a presentation, you people are the best kind of people. So many of you are on my list. Thank you for loving me at my worst and celebrating the small victories.

Lastly, to my little family. You are the bravest crew and the reason I live. This journey has been toughest on you and yet you continue to treat me like you always have. I carry your strength with me every day in hopes that one day I can pay it forward. Thank you for filling my cup (proverbially and literally) daily and for sacred snuggles. I love you past heaven.

Made in the USA
Monee, IL
24 May 2022